DRCOG Revision Guide

Nigel Davies and Paul Hodges

DRCOG Revision Guide

A guide to success in the new-style examination

Published by the RCOG Press at the
Royal College of Obstetricians and Gynaecologists
27 Sussex Place, Regent's Park, London NW1 4RG

Registered Charity No. 213280

RCOG Press Editor Jane Moody

Indexing by Liza Furnival,
Medical Indexing Ltd

Text designed & typeset at the
Typographic Design Unit

Printed in the United Kingdom by
Latimer Trend & Co. Ltd

Contents

Foreword

Modern professional practice, be it in medicine, law, education or accountancy requires evidence of attainment of competence. We need to demonstrate to our patients, customers, clients and colleagues that we are who we say we are and that we are capable of delivering a high-quality service in our chosen field. Paper qualifications have never carried more weight, nor been regarded more highly than in the cynical world of the 21st century. The corollary to this statement is that the qualifications themselves must only be awarded after a comprehensive and rigorous assessment of the knowledge of the candidate. This pressure for validation of quality has driven the RCOG to perform radical surgery on its examinations, both for the Membership and the Diploma of this College. Much has been learned from educational theory and from the format and structure of other examinations both within and outside the world of medicine. Some of the changes have been driven by wider manipulations of the structure of medical training in UK, for example the move away from 6-month attachments in obstetrics and gynaecology at senior house officer level for the majority of aspiring GPs. However, there is a higher motivation to the process of change within the RCOG's examinations, namely to make our processes more fair, more transparent and more 'fit for purpose' for the next decade. The role of the GP in women's health has moved a long distance from the provision of home delivery towards a more team-based and holistic model of care. Moves to provide more services in general practice and away from the hospital setting have placed a greater burden on the GP, particularly in the areas of benign gynaecology and sexual health, and the new curriculum and syllabus for DRCOG reflects this.

The DRCOG has always been a voluntary examination. It sits alongside the qualifications provided by the Royal College of General Practitioners and offers the trainee with special interest in a non-hospital-based practice in women's health a means of developing a more specialised knowledge base. The DRCOG cannot test the candidate's ability to perform practical procedures or to counsel women in a sympathetic and informative way. These skills can only properly be judged within the workplace by repeated interaction with a competent trainer. General practice has always excelled at this aspect of training and assessment and we are confident that those who complete GP training in UK and who hold the DRCOG will be seen as able and efficient practitioners who can support their female patients through the myriad of health needs and disease pathways that populate the field of women's health. Those of us who practice full time in this area do so because of our fascination with reproductive medicine and the privilege of participating in this most deeply meaningful and professionally rewarding area of medical practice. In updating and improving the DRCOG, we hope to maintain high standards in primary care and to transmit some of our enthusiasm to colleagues in general practice.

Professor William L Ledger FRCOG
Chairman, Examination and Assessment Committee
Royal College of Obstetricians and Gynaecologists

About the authors

Nigel Davies is a Consultant Obstetrician and Gynaecologist at the University Hospital of Wales, Cardiff. He is active in postgraduate education and assessment, having recently been a College Tutor. He has been closely involved with the DRCOG examination for over 10 years and for the past 4 years has been the Chair of the DRCOG Sub-committee.

Paul Hodges has worked in the Examination Department of the College since 2003 and has been Deputy to the Head of the Department since April 2006. From 2000 to 2003, he worked in a similar capacity at the Institute of Healthcare Management. He completed a part-time PhD in First World War history in 2007 and is hoping to publish a resultant book soon. This is his third book for the RCOG Press and he is active in assessment and medical education research and publication.

Acknowledgements

We would like to thank our families for their forbearance in adding to our workloads with authorship. Their love and support means everything to us.

We would like to thank Dr Michael Murphy, Director of Education, Royal College of Obstetricians and Gynaecologists, for his continuing inspiration and vision in this area, and for his substantial help with the text of this book. We would also like to thank Professor William Ledger, Chair of the Examinations and Assessment Committee, Royal College of Obstetricians and Gynaecologists, for his support and for writing the Foreword to this book.

Finally, we also would like to acknowledge the outstanding effort of the present and past members of the Diploma Committee and Diploma Working Group in enabling the new and improved examination to take place.

Nigel Davies
Paul Hodges

Abbreviations

ACE	angiotensin-converting enzyme
BCG	bacille Calmette-Guérin
BP	blood pressure
BOF	best of five question
CTG	cardiotocograph
DHEAS	dehydroepiandrosterone sulphate
DMPA	depot medroxyprogesterone acetate
DRCOG	Diploma of the Royal College of Obstetricians and Gynaecologists
DXA	dual-energy X-ray absorptiometry
EMQ	extended matching question
FISH	fluorescence in situ hybridisation
FSH	follicle-stimulating hormone
GMC	General Medical Council
GnRH	gonadotrophin-releasing hormone
GP	general practitioner
hCG	human chorionic gonadotrophin
HIV	human immunodeficiency virus
HPV	human papillomavirus
IUCD	intrauterine contraceptive device
LH	luteinising hormone

MCH	corpuscular haemoglobin
MCHC	corpuscular haemoglobin concentration
MCQ	multiple choice question
MCV	mean corpuscular volume
MI	myocardial infarction
MMR	measles, mumps and rubella
OSCE	objective structured clinical examination
PMETB	Postgraduate Medical Education and Training Board
POP	progestogen-only pill
RCOG	Royal College of Obstetricians and Gynaecologists
RhD	rhesus factor
SBA	single best answer question
SSRI	selective serotonin reuptake inhibitor
T_4	thyroxine
TB	tuberculosis
TSH	thyroid-stimulating hormone

1 | Introduction

The Diploma examination of the Royal College of Obstetricians and Gynaecologists (hereafter referred to by its common acronym: DRCOG) is designed for UK-based general practitioners (hereafter GP or GPs). Although suitable for supporting GPs' general medical knowledge and practice, the DRCOG is particularly useful for GPs wishing to offer obstetric, gynaecological and other aspects of women's healthcare in a primary healthcare setting, such as GP surgeries, walk-in centres and family-planning clinics. The DRCOG is not a mandatory qualification but it remains popular as evidence that Diplomates have an interest and some skill in the specialty. In addition, the DRCOG has a value in helping Diplomates to find good GP posts or partnerships. However, it must be emphasised that the DRCOG is not a specialist qualification and it is not relevant to competition for specialist training posts in obstetrics and gynaecology. More widely for the College, the DRCOG aims to support the College's core mission of 'Setting standards to improve women's health'. It is of paramount importance that women and unborn babies receive accurate, sensitive and skilled care from their GPs. The DRCOG examination therefore plays a vital role in setting and maintaining standards in this key area of primary care.

Prior to October 2007, the format of the DRCOG examination had been unchanged since the early 1990s when the RCOG introduced an objective structured clinical examination (OSCE) component. This was the RCOG's first use of an OSCE in its postgraduate examinations. However, since the early 1990s there have been many developments in examination techniques and question types, several of which have been incorporated into the College's Membership examinations. From October 2007, the DRCOG examination will also benefit from the experience of these innovations.

From January 2005 to February 2006, a College working group looked closely at many aspects of the current DRCOG qualification and highlighted the need for reform in certain areas. Therefore, in 2006, the previous short and not very well structured syllabus was replaced by a new, properly structured curriculum and multidimensional syllabus. This work has received the full approval of the Postgraduate Medical Education and Training Board (PMETB), although examinations like the DRCOG do not currently fall within PMETB's remit. In addition, in February 2006, the College removed the 6-month training requirement in hospital-based obstetrics and gynaecology for Diploma candidates wishing to use the DRCOG postnominals. Thereafter, all candidates who pass the DRCOG have been enrolled as Diplomates of the College and are permitted to use the postnominals. This change was necessary because following the recent reorganisation of postgraduate medical training 6-month rotations at senior house officer level have generally been replaced by 4-month blocks of experience. Moreover, it is also theoretically possible for doctors in the Foundation Year of training to attempt the DRCOG examination. Indeed, with the removal of the training requirement entirely, some candidates may be tempted to sit the examination without any in-depth experience of obstetrics and gynaecology, armed only with 'book knowledge'. However, the College hopes that the numbers of these candidates will be low and the authors would discourage such candidates from attempting the examination. On the other hand, the College intends that the new examination will perform well as an effective competency-based assessment and would encourage all suitably qualified candidates to apply.

The new curriculum and syllabus reflect the current concept that the DRCOG is an assessment of knowledge, skills and attitudes as applied to women's health, as practised by the GPs in the UK and also the expectation that at least 3 months' training in the subject has been completed. Nonetheless, a serious challenge for the remodelled DRCOG will remain in continuing to run successfully as an effective assessment of clinical knowledge and competence, without extensive workplace-based training for candidates being in place. With this in mind, issues of validity and reliability – the heartbeat of educational and evaluative benefits – will be key.

With the removal of the training requirement, and in the context of a reorganised postgraduate medical training programme, the challenge for the RCOG has been to set a new examination in women's health that is up-to-date and relevant to GP trainees and also an effective assessment of the DRCOG curriculum and syllabus. This has been achieved using a combination of multiple choice questions (MCQs), 'best of five' questions (also referred to as 'single best answer' questions) and extended matching questions (EMQs). It is our hope that this book will guide those attempting the new-style DRCOG through the examination and will allow doctors with an interest in women's health, and particularly UK-based GPs, to certificate their interest and knowledge in this core subject of family practice.

2 | The curriculum

The RCOG takes the view that the DRCOG should be a certificate of appropriate knowledge of women's health care as applied to the GP in the UK and this view is reflected in the new DRCOG curriculum and syllabus.

The old-style DRCOG examination was not derived from an explicit curriculum. However, the previous DRCOG syllabus, in use from the early 1990s onwards, was vast and effectively meant that candidates were required to understand all aspects of obstetrics and gynaecology, neonatology, genitourinary medicine and contraception. The new curriculum and syllabus have narrowed those domains of knowledge to those areas of women's health appropriate to a UK-based GP. For example, you are no longer expected to know how to perform a hysterectomy but you would be expected to be able to counsel a woman with regard to the complications associated with a hysterectomy and the relative benefits of choosing other options for the management of menorrhagia.

Candidates applying for the DRCOG examination should note that, with effect from October 2007, the DRCOG examination will be subject to a new curriculum and syllabus. The new DRCOG will measure the candidate's ability to apply knowledge in relation to common and important aspects of women's health, as outlined in the syllabus, and to make appropriate clinical judgements.

The curriculum defines all those related domains that make up the complete knowledge set, skills and attitudes expected of DRCOG candidates. The curriculum presented here is correct at the time of publication but may change with time. The most up-to-date version of the curriculum will be available on the RCOG website (www.rcog.org.uk).

The curriculum is divided into seven modules:

▶ Module 1: Basic clinical skills
▶ Module 2: Basic surgical skills and surgical procedures
▶ Module 3: Antenatal care
▶ Module 4: Management of labour and delivery
▶ Module 5: Postpartum problems (the puerperium) including
　　　　　　neonatal problems

5

▶ Module 6: Gynaecological problems
▶ Module 7: Contraception and termination of pregnancy

MODULE 1: BASIC CLINICAL SKILLS

Learning outcomes

To understand and demonstrate the appropriate knowledge, skills and attitudes to perform specialist assessment of patients by means of clinical history taking and physical examination. To manage problems effectively, and to communicate well with patients, relatives and colleagues in a variety of clinical situations. To demonstrate effective time management. To be aware of the legal and ethical issues relating to medical certification and the status of the unborn child.

History taking

Knowledge criteria
▶ Define the patterns of symptoms in patients presenting with obstetric and gynaecological problems.

Clinical competency
▶ Take and analyse an obstetric and gynaecological history in a succinct and logical manner.
▶ Manage difficulties of language, physical and mental impairment.
▶ Use interpreters and health advocates appropriately.

Professional skills and attitudes
▶ Show empathy and develop rapport with patients.
▶ Appreciate the importance of psychological factors for patients and their relatives.
▶ Be aware of the interaction of social factors with the patient's illness.
▶ Demonstrate an awareness of the impact of health problems on the ability to function at work.

Clinical examination and investigation

Knowledge criteria
► Understand the pathophysiological basis of physical signs.
► Understand the indications, risks, benefits and effectiveness of investigations

Clinical competency
► Perform a reliable and appropriate examination, including:
  ▷ abdominal examination (nonpregnant and pregnant)
  ▷ vaginal examination (bimanual, Cuscoe speculum)
  ▷ microbiology swabs (vagina, cervix, urethra)
  ▷ cervical smear
► Perform investigations competently where relevant.
► Interpret the results of investigations.
► Liaise and discuss investigations with colleagues.

Professional skills and attitudes
► Respect patients' dignity and confidentiality.
► Acknowledge and respect cultural diversity.
► Involve relatives appropriately.
► Appreciate the need for a chaperone.
► Provide explanations to patients.

Training support
► General Medical Council. Good Medical Practice.
► Royal College of Obstetricians and Gynaecologists. *Maintaining Good Medical Practice in Obstetrics and Gynaecology: the Role of the RCOG.* London: RCOG; 1999.
► *GynaecologicalExaminations: Guidelines for Specialist Practice.* London: RCOG; 2002.

Note keeping

Knowledge criteria
► Understand the importance and conventions of accurate clinical note keeping.

7

► Know the relevance of data protection pertaining to patient confidentiality.
► Freedom of Information Act and its implications.

Clinical competency
► Record and communicate concisely, accurately, legibly and confidentially, the results of the history, examination, investigations, differential diagnosis and management plan.
► Mark each note entry with date, signature, name and status.

Professional skills and attitudes
► Appreciate the importance of timely dictation, cost effective use of medical secretaries and increasing use of electronic communication.
► Communicate promptly and accurately with primary care and other agencies.
► Demonstrate courtesy towards secretaries,

Training support
► Caldicott Committee. *Report on the Review of Patient-Identifiable Information.* London: Department of Health; 1997.

Legal issues relating to medical certification

Knowledge criteria
► Know the legal responsibilities of completing maternity, birth, sickness and death certificates.
► Awareness of the Confidential Enquiry into Maternal and Child Health (CEMACH).

Clinical competency
► Complete relevant medical certification.

Professional skills and attitudes
► Obtain suitable evidence or know who to consult.

Training support
► CEMACH reports [www.cemach.org.uk].
► Royal College of Obstetricians and Gynaecologists. *Registration of Stillbirths and Certification for Pregnancy Loss before 24 Weeks of Gestation.* Good Practice No. 4. London: RCOG; 2005.
► General Medical Council. *0–18 years: Guidance for all Doctors.* London: GMC; 2007 [www.gmc-uk.org/guidance/archive/GMC_0-18.pdf].

Time management and decision making

Knowledge criteria
► Understand clinical priorities.

Clinical competency
► Prioritise tasks.
► Work with increasing efficiency as clinical skills develop.
► Know when to get help.
► Anticipate future clinical events and plan appropriately.

Professional skills and attitudes
► Have realistic expectations of tasks to be completed and timeframe for tasks.
► Be willing to consult and work as part of a team.
► Learn to be flexible, be willing to take advice and change in the light of new information.

Communication

Knowledge criteria
► Understand the components of effective verbal and nonverbal communication.

Clinical competency
► Demonstrate listening skills.
► Use open questions where possible.
► Give appropriate information in a manner that patients and

9

relatives understand and assess their comprehension.
- ▶ Communicate clearly both verbally and in writing to patients, including those whose first language may not be English.
- ▶ Give clear information and feedback and share communication with patients and relatives.
- ▶ Break bad news sensitively.

Professional skills and attitudes
- ▶ Demonstrate ability to:
  - ▷ involve patients in decision making
  - ▷ offer choices
  - ▷ respect patients' views
  - ▷ use appropriate nonverbal communication.

Training support
- ▶ Royal College of Obstetricians and Gynaecologists. Patient information [www.rcog.org.uk/index.asp?PageID=625].
- ▶ Sands [www.uk-sands.org] guidance for professionals.

Ethics and legal issues

Knowledge criteria
- ▶ Be aware of the implications of the legal status of the unborn child.
- ▶ Understand appropriateness of consent to postmortem examination.

Clinical competency
- ▶ Use written material correctly and accurately.
- ▶ Gain valid consent from patients.
- ▶ Discuss clinical risk.

Professional skills and attitudes
- ▶ Give appropriate information in a manner that patients and relatives understand and assess their comprehension.
- ▶ Be aware of the patient's needs as an individual.
- ▶ Respect diversity.

Training support
► Royal College of Obstetricians and Gynaecologists. Consent Advice Series [www.rcog.org.uk/index.asp?PageID=686].
► Royal College of Obstetricians and Gynaecologists. *Law and Ethics in Relation to Court-authorised Obstetric Intervention.* Ethics Committee Guideline No. 1. London: RCOG; 2006.

MODULE 2: BASIC SURGICAL SKILLS AND SURGICAL PROCEDURES

Learning outcomes

To understand and demonstrate appropriate knowledge, skills and attitudes in relation to basic surgical skills and surgical procedures.

Knowledge criteria
► Legal issues around consent to surgical procedures, including consent of minors, adults with incapacity and adults and children in emergency situations.
► An understanding of the general anatomical relationship of the pelvic organs.
► Complications of O&G surgery.
► Commonly encountered infections, including an understanding of the principles of infection control.
► Appropriate use of blood and blood products.

Clinical competency
► Interpret preoperative investigations.
► Arrange preoperative management.
► Explain procedures to patient.
► Advise patient on postoperative course.

Professional skills and attitudes
► Recognise and initiate collaboration with other disciplines, before and after surgery.
► Recognise that decision making is a collaborative process between doctor and patient.

Training support
► Royal College of Obstetricians and Gynaecologists. Consent Advice Series [www.rcog.org.uk/index.asp?PageID=686].

Surgical procedures

Knowledge criteria
► Complications of surgery including:
  ▷ deep vein thrombosis/pulmonary embolism
  ▷ infection (wound, urinary tract, respiratory, intra-abdominal and pelvic)
  ▷ primary and secondary haemorrhage (intraoperative and postoperative)
  ▷ characteristics, recognition, prevention, eradication and pathological effects of all commonly encountered bacteria, and viruses specific to O&G surgery.

Clinical competency
► Observe common gynaecological procedures including:
  ▷ marsupialisation of Bartholin's abscess
  ▷ evacuation of retained products
  ▷ diagnostic laparoscopy
  ▷ diagnostic hysteroscopy
  ▷ minor cervical procedures
  ▷ excision/biopsy of vulval lesions
  ▷ surgical treatment for ectopic pregnancy
  ▷ hysterectomy
  ▷ prolapse procedures
  ▷ endometrial ablation.

Postoperative care

Knowledge criteria
► Postoperative complications related to obstetric and gynaecological procedures.

Clinical competency
► Make appropriate postoperative plans of management.
► Conduct appropriate review of:
  ▷ fluid/electrolyte balance
  ▷ catheter management.
► Manage complications including wound, thromboembolism and infection.

Professional skills and attitudes
► Select and undertake relevant postoperative investigations.
► Construct an appropriate discharge letter.

Training support
► Royal College of Obstetricians and Gynaecologists. *Thromboprophylaxis During Pregnancy, Labour and after Vaginal Delivery*. Green-top Guideline No. 37. London: RCOG; 2004.
► Scottish Intercollegiate Guidelines Network. *Prophylaxis of Venous Thromboembolism*. SIGN Guideline No. 62. Edinburgh: SIGN; 2004.

MODULE 3: ANTENATAL CARE

Learning outcomes

To understand and demonstrate appropriate knowledge, skills and attitudes in relation to antenatal care and maternal complications of pregnancy.

Knowledge criteria
► Periconceptional care.
► Purposes and practice of antenatal care.
► Management of normal and complicated pregnancy, birth and puerperium.
► Genetic modes of inheritance, common genetic conditions and the diagnosis thereof.
► Recognition of domestic violence.
► Problems of pregnancy at extremes of reproductive age.
► Awareness of drug and alcohol abuse.
► Knowledge of common disorders of pregnancy including:

- $\triangleright$ hypertension
- $\triangleright$ urinary tract infection, pyelonephritis
- $\triangleright$ varicose veins
- $\triangleright$ anaemia
- $\triangleright$ heart disease
- $\triangleright$ cholestasis
- $\triangleright$ diabetes
- $\triangleright$ thyroid dysfunction
- $\triangleright$ inflammatory bowel disease
- $\triangleright$ asthma and tuberculosis
- $\triangleright$ psychological/psychiatric disorders
- $\triangleright$ symphysis pubis dysfunction
- $\triangleright$ epilepsy, multiple sclerosis, migraine
- $\triangleright$ HIV, hepatitis, syphilis, rubella, varicella
- $\triangleright$ issues relevant to a migrant population.

Clinical competency
- ▶ Conduct a booking visit.
- ▶ Conduct follow-up visits.
- ▶ Arrange appropriate investigations.
- ▶ Participate in the management of:
  - $\triangleright$ fetal growth restriction
  - $\triangleright$ multiple pregnancy
  - $\triangleright$ antepartum haemorrhage
  - $\triangleright$ malpresentation
  - $\triangleright$ preterm prelabour rupture of the fetal membranes
  - $\triangleright$ hypertension in pregnancy
  - $\triangleright$ post-dates pregnancy.
- ▶ Participate in the diagnosis and management of the conditions listed above in *Knowledge criteria*.

Professional skills and attitudes
- ▶ Liaise with midwives and other health professionals to optimise patient management.
- ▶ Empower and inform women to make appropriate choices for themselves and their families in pregnancy and childbirth.
- ▶ Explain correctly and place in context for the patient:

▷ principles of screening for structural defects, chromosomal abnormalities haemoglobinopathies

▷ effects upon fetus and neonate of common infections during pregnancy.

▶ Liaise effectively with colleagues in other disciplines, clinical and nonclinical.

Training support

▶ Workplace-based experience:

▷ attendance at local perinatal morbidity and mortality meetings

▷ risk assessment meetings.

MODULE 4: MANAGEMENT OF LABOUR AND DELIVERY

Learning outcomes

▶ To understand and demonstrate appropriate knowledge, skills and attitudes in relation to labour and delivery.

Labour

Knowledge criteria

▶ Mechanisms of normal labour and delivery.

▶ Induction and augmentation of labour.

▶ Drugs acting upon the myometrium.

▶ Structure and use of partograms.

▶ Fluid balance in labour.

▶ Regional anaesthesia, analgesia and sedation.

▶ Fetal wellbeing and compromise.

▶ Prolonged labour.

▶ Emergency policies/maternal collapse/haemorrhage.

▶ Preterm labour/premature rupture of membranes.

▶ Multiple pregnancy in labour.

▶ Severe pre-eclampsia and eclampsia.

▶ Interpretation of CTG.

▶ In utero fetal death , including legal issues.

Clinical competency
▶ Participate in the labour ward management of:
  ▷ induction of labour
  ▷ women with prolonged labour
  ▷ women with a previous caesarean section
  ▷ preterm labour
  ▷ women with an abnormal CTG
  ▷ acute resuscitation.

Professional skills and attitudes
▶ Respect cultural/religious differences in attitudes to childbirth.
▶ Liaise effectively with colleagues in other disciplines, clinical and Nonclinical.

Training support
▶ CTG training.
▶ Eclampsia drill.
▶ Drill for obstetrical collapse.
▶ Perinatal mortality and morbidity meetings.
▶ RCOG guidelines [www.rcog.org.uk].
▶ Sands [www.uk-sands.org] guidance for professionals.

Delivery

Knowledge criteria
▶ Normal vaginal delivery.
▶ Operative vaginal delivery.
▶ Caesarean section.
▶ Regional anaesthesia.

Clinical competency
▶ Ability to discuss the procedures in the knowledge criteria in the light of personal observation.

Professional skills and attitudes
▶ Awareness of emotional implications for the woman, her family and hospital staff.
▶ Supporting women in appropriate decision making in choice of delivery.

Training support
▶ Perinatal mortality and morbidity meetings.
▶ Labour ward guidelines.
▶ CEMACH reports.

MODULE 5: POSTPARTUM PROBLEMS (THE PUERPERIUM) INCLUDING NEONATAL PROBLEMS

Learning outcomes

To understand and demonstrate appropriate knowledge, skills and attitudes in relation to postpartum maternal and neonatal problems.

Knowledge criteria
▶ Normal and abnormal postpartum period.
▶ Postpartum haemorrhage.
▶ Perineal care.
▶ Postpartum depression and psychosis.
▶ Infant feeding and breast problems.
▶ Thromboembolism.
▶ Contraception.
▶ Sepsis.

Clinical competency
▶ Participate in the management of:
  ▷ the normal puerperium, including contraception
  ▷ breast problems
  ▷ puerperal psychological disorders
  ▷ perineal and vaginal tears
  ▷ postpartum sepsis
  ▷ postpartum haemorrhage.

Professional skills and attitudes
- ► Understand the roles of other healthcare professionals; such as midwives, social workers, psychiatrists, physiotherapists.
- ► Display empathy with women and their families where puerperal problems arise.

Training support
- ► National Childbirth Trust [www.nctpregnancyandbabycare.com].
- ► MIND (National Association for Mental Health) [www.mind.org.uk].
- ► RCOG guidelines [www.rcog.org.uk].

NEONATAL PROBLEMS

Learning outcomes

To understand and demonstrate appropriate knowledge, skills and attitudes in relation to neonatal problems.

Knowledge criteria
- ► Knowledge of first day neonatal examination.
- ► Resuscitation of the newborn.
- ► Neonatal jaundice.

Clinical competency
- ► Neonatal resuscitation.

Professional skills and attitudes
- ► Liaise with paediatricians and the neonatal team.

Training support
- ► Perinatal morbidity and mortality meetings.
- ► Neonatal resuscitation training.

MODULE 6: GYNAECOLOGICAL PROBLEMS

Learning outcomes

To understand and demonstrate appropriate knowledge, skills and attitudes in relation to common gynaecological problems including subfertility, early pregnancy loss, urogynaecology and oncology.

Benign gynaecology

Knowledge criteria
▶ Knowledge of common disorders including the following:
  ▷ abnormal genital tract bleeding
  ▷ polycystic ovary syndrome
  ▷ the climacteric
  ▷ pelvic pain
  ▷ vaginal discharge
  ▷ pelvic inflammatory disease
  ▷ delayed puberty
  ▷ issues relevant to a migrant population.

Clinical competency
▶ Diagnose, investigate and participate in the management of common gynaecological disorders.

Professional skills and attitudes
▶ Counsel patients about the options available.
▶ Liaise with colleagues in other disciplines where required.

Training support
▶ RCOG guidelines[www.rcog.org.uk/index.asp?PageID=8].
▶ Attendance at genitourinary clinics.

Sexually transmitted infections

Knowledge criteria
▶ Knowledge of common disorders including:

▷ chlamydia
  ▷ gonorrhoea
  ▷ syphilis
  ▷ HIV
  ▷ herpes
  ▷ Trichomonas
  ▷ HPV
  ▷ hepatitis.

Clinical competency
► Diagnose, investigate and participate in the management of the listed sexually transmitted infections.
► Understand the principles of contact tracing.

Professional skills and attitudes
► Counsel patients about the options available.
► Liaise with colleagues in other disciplines where required.
► Be aware of confidentiality issues.

Training support
► RCOG guidelines.
► Attendance at genitourinary clinics.
► British Association for Sexual Health and HIV [www.bashh.org].

Subfertility

Knowledge criteria
► Knowledge of common disorders leading to male and female subfertility:
  ▷ basic investigations and treatment of the subfertile couple
  ▷ principles of assisted conception.

Clinical competency
► Take a history from the couple with subfertility.
► Initiate basic investigation of male and female infertility.
► Counsel about management options.

Professional skills and attitudes
► Appreciate the importance of psychological factors for patients and

their partners.
► Acknowledge cultural issues, especially with respect to use of gametes.
► Liaise effectively with colleagues in secondary and tertiary referral.

Training support
► Attendance at subfertility clinics.
► Useful websites:
  ▷ Royal College of Obstetricians and Gynaecologists
    [www.rcog.org.uk]
  ▷ National Institute for Health and Clinical Excellence
    [www.nice.org.uk]
  ▷ Human Fertilisation and Embryology Authority [www.hfea.gov.uk].

Early pregnancy loss

Knowledge criteria
► Knowledge of clinical features, investigation and management of
  common disorders leading to early pregnancy loss:
  ▷ miscarriage (including recurrent)
  ▷ ectopic pregnancy
  ▷ molar pregnancy.

Clinical competency
► Clinical assessment of miscarriage and ectopic pregnancy.
► Participate in the medical and surgical management of miscarriage
  and ectopic pregnancy.
► Counsel about management options.

Professional skills and attitudes
► Appreciate importance of psychological factors with relation to
  pregnancy loss.
► Recognise high-risk clinical situation and manage appropriately.
► Communicate effectively and sensitively with patients and family.

Training support
► Royal College of Obstetricians and Gynaecologists. *The Management
  of Early Pregnancy Loss*. Green-top Guideline No. 25. London: RCOG;
  2006.

- Support-group literature.
- Attendance at early pregnancy assessment unit/clinic.

Urogynaecology and pelvic floor problems

Knowledge criteria
- Knowledge of clinical features, investigation and management of common disorders of the female urogenital tract:
  - urinary infection
  - urinary and faecal incontinence
  - urogenital prolapse.

Clinical competency
- Take a urogynaecological history.
- Diagnose and treat urinary tract infections.
- Initiate nonsurgical treatment of prolapse and urinary incontinence.

Professional skills and attitudes
- Appreciate the importance of psychological factors.
- Deal sensitively with issues regarding incontinence.
- Explain actions, complications and adverse effects of common drug treatments.

Training support
- Attendance at clinics dealing with patients presenting with urinary incontinence and urogenital prolapse.
- Useful websites:
  - www.nice.org.uk
  - www.sign.org.uk.

Oncology

Knowledge criteria
- Knowledge of clinical features, investigation and management of premalignant and malignant conditions of the female genital tract:

- ▷ vulva
- ▷ cervix
- ▷ endometrium
- ▷ ovary.
- ► Indications and limitations of screening for malignant disease:
  - ▷ cervical cytology
  - ▷ ultrasound
  - ▷ genetics
  - ▷ biochemistry.
- ► Understanding of the options available for palliative and terminal care:
  - ▷ relief of symptoms
  - ▷ community support.

Clinical competency
- ► Perform a cervical smear and counsel about cytology reports.
- ► Ability to counsel a patient for colposcopy.

Professional skills and attitudes
- ► Explain cytology reports clearly and sensitively to patients and relatives.
- ► Appreciate the importance of psychological factors for patients and their families.
- ► Liaise with colleagues in allied disciplines.
- ► Deal sensitively with issues regarding palliative care and death.
- ► Acknowledge cultural issues, especially with respect to death and burial practices.

Training support
- ► Attendance at colposcopy clinics.
- ► Useful website: British Society for Colposcopy and Cervical Pathology [www.bsccp.org.uk].

MODULE 7: CONTRACEPTION AND TERMINATION OF PREGNANCY

Learning outcomes

To understand and demonstrate appropriate knowledge, skills and attitudes in relation to fertility control (contraception and termination of pregnancy).

(There may be conscientious objection to the acquisition of certain skills.)

Knowledge criteria
- ▶ Indications, contraindications, complications, mode of action and efficacy of contraceptive methods.
- ▶ The law relating to fertility control, termination of pregnancy, consent and the Sexual Offences Act 2003.
- ▶ Methods available for termination of pregnancy.

Clinical competency
- ▶ Take a history in relation to:
  - ▷ contraceptive and sexual health needs and risk assessment
  - ▷ unplanned pregnancy.
- ▶ Counsel about:
  - ▷ contraceptive options
  - ▷ emergency contraception
  - ▷ unplanned pregnancy options
  - ▷ sterilisation procedures.
- ▶ Deliver hormonal methods of contraception.
- ▶ Deliver hormonal emergency contraception.

Professional skills and attitudes
- ▶ Counsel patients sensitively about the options available and associated sexual health issues.
- ▶ Respect the patient's right to confidentiality.
- ▶ Explain clearly and openly treatments, complications and adverse effects of drug treatment.
- ▶ Liaise effectively with colleagues in other disciplines, clinical and nonclinical.

24

► Respect cultural and religious diversity and beliefs.

Training support
► Family planning sessions/genitourinary medicine clinics.
► Use of training models.
► Medical Foundation for AIDS & Sexual Health. *Recommended Standards for Sexual Health Services* London: MFASH; 2005 [www.medfash.org.uk].
► British Medical Association. The Laws and Ethics of Abortion: BMA views (March 1997, revised December 1999 [www.bma.org.uk/ap.nsf/content/abortion].
► General Medical Council. *0–18 years: Guidance for all Doctors.* London: GMC; 2007 [www.gmc-uk.org/guidance/archive/GMC_0-18.pdf].
► Useful websites:
  ▷ Royal College of Obstetricians and Gynaecologists [www.rcog.org.uk]
  ▷ National Institute for Health and Clinical Excellence [www.nice.org.uk]
  ▷ Faculty of Sexual and Reproductive Healthcare [www.fsrh.org.uk]
  ▷ Medical Foundation for AIDS & Sexual Health [www.medfash.org.uk].

3 | The syllabus

The syllabus is an outline of the main points of the curriculum and is designed to aid your learning for the DRCOG examination. The syllabus is correct at the time of publication but may change with time. An updated version of the syllabus will be available on the RCOG website (www.rcog.org.uk)

The syllabus is also divided into seven modules based upon the curriculum.

Module 1: Basic clinical skills

You will be expected to understand the patterns of symptoms in women presenting with obstetric problems, gynaecological problems, sexually transmitted infections and patients in a family planning setting.

You will be expected to demonstrate an understanding of the pathophysiological basis of physical signs and understand the indications, risks, benefits and effectiveness of investigations in a clinical setting.

You will be required to demonstrate an understanding of the components of effective verbal and nonverbal communication.

You will need to be aware of relevant ethical and legal issues including the implications of the legal status of the unborn child, the legal issues relating to medical certification and issues related to medical confidentiality. You will be expected to understand the issues surrounding consent in all clinical situations including postmortem examination and termination of pregnancy.

Module 2: Basic surgical skills

You will be expected to demonstrate an understanding of commonly performed obstetric and gynaecological surgical procedures, including their complications and the legal issues around consent to surgical procedures. You will need to be aware of commonly encountered infections, including an understanding of the principles of infection control.

You will be expected to interpret preoperative investigations and be aware of the principles involved in appropriate preoperative and postoperative care.

Module 3: Antenatal care

You will be expected to understand and demonstrate appropriate knowledge and attitudes in relation to periconceptional care, antenatal care and maternal complications of pregnancy. The examiners will expect you to be aware of antenatal strategies for problem prevention and be conversant with effective and appropriate lifestyle advice with regard to substance misuse, psychiatric illness, problems of pregnancy at extremes of reproductive age and issues of domestic violence. An appreciation of emotional issues and cultural awareness is expected.

You will be expected to have a good understanding of common medical disorders and the effect that pregnancy may have on them, and also their effect, in turn, upon the pregnancy. Knowledge of therapeutics in antenatal care is expected. You will be expected to demonstrate your ability to assess and manage these conditions. You will need to show understanding of the roles of other professionals, the importance of liaison and empathic teamwork.

You will be expected to understand the principles of antenatal screening, including screening for structural defects, chromosomal abnormalities and haemoglobinopathies and the effects upon fetus and neonate of relevant infections during pregnancy.

Module 4: Management of labour and delivery

You will be expected to have the knowledge, understanding and judgement to be capable of initial management of intrapartum problems in a hospital and in a community setting. This will include: knowledge and understanding of normal and abnormal labour, data and investigation interpretation, induction and augmentation of labour, assessment of fetal wellbeing and compromise.

An understanding of the management of all obstetric emergencies is expected. You will need to demonstrate appropriate knowledge of regional anaesthesia, analgesia and operative delivery including caesarean section. You will need to be able to demonstrate respect for cultural and religious differences in attitudes to childbirth.

Module 5: Postpartum problems (the puerperium) including neonatal problems

You will be expected to understand and demonstrate appropriate knowledge, management skills and attitudes in relation to postpartum maternal problems including: the normal and abnormal postpartum period, postpartum haemorrhage, therapeutics, perineal care, psychological disorders, infant feeding and breast problems.

You will be expected to demonstrate an understanding of the investigation and management of immediate neonatal problems including neonatal resuscitation.

Module 6: Gynaecological problems

You will be expected to demonstrate appropriate knowledge, management skills and attitudes in relation to benign gynaecological problems including: urogynaecology, paediatric and adolescent gynaecology, endocrine problems, pelvic pain and abnormal vaginal bleeding.

This will include knowledge of early pregnancy loss, including clinical features, investigation and management of disorders leading to early pregnancy loss: miscarriage (including recurrent), ectopic pregnancy and molar pregnancy.

You will be expected to demonstrate an ability to assess and manage common sexually transmitted infections, including HIV/AIDS, and be familiar with their modes of transmission and clinical features. You will be expected to understand the principles of contact tracing. You will also be expected to know the basis of national screening programmes and their local implementation through local care pathways.

You will be expected to demonstrate appropriate knowledge of clinical features, investigation and management of premalignant and malignant conditions of the female genital tract. You will be expected to have an understanding of the indications and limitations of screening for premalignant and malignant disease. An understanding of the options available for palliative and terminal care including relief of symptoms and community support will be expected.

The examiners will expect you to demonstrate appropriate knowledge and attitudes in relation to subfertility. This includes an understanding of

29

the epidemiology, aetiology, management and prognosis of male and female fertility problems. You will be expected to have a broad based knowledge of investigation and management of the infertile couple in a primary care setting and appropriate knowledge of assisted reproductive techniques including and the legal and ethical implications of these procedures.

Module 7: Fertility control (contraception and termination of pregnancy)

You will be expected to demonstrate appropriate knowledge, management skills and attitudes in relation to fertility control and termination of pregnancy. You will be expected to understand the indications, contraindications, complications, mode of action and efficacy of all reversible and irreversible contraceptive methods. You will be expected to demonstrate appropriate knowledge of abortion and should be familiar with the accompanying laws related to abortion, consent, child protection and the Sexual Offences Act(s).

There may be conscientious objection to the acquisition of certain skills in areas of sexual and reproductive health but knowledge and appropriate attitudes as described above will be expected.

4 | The new DRCOG examination

The new curriculum and syllabus will clearly drive forward the formative usage of the DRCOG in combination with the changes to GP training brought in under the Modernising Medical Careers initiative. Key to this will be 'blueprinting' of the examination (Figure 1). This is a method of checking that each examination question is categorised by what it aims to test, and the examination blueprint thus provides an overall picture of the entire examination's coverage. The aim is to ensure that the examination is testing as much of the syllabus as possible, with minimal duplication of testing the same domain of knowledge in the different question types.

Standard setting

Since April 2006, the DRCOG examination has had a pass mark that has been standard set. Standard setting is an acknowledgement that some multiple choice, single best answer ('best of five') and extended matching format questions are more difficult than others. Therefore, a different pass mark is used for each examination, depending on the overall difficulty of that examination. Pass marks will thus fluctuate and the RCOG has no fixed or predetermined quota of candidates that it aims to pass or fail. A panel of representative consultants and GPs implements the standard setting procedures for the DRCOG examination. The standard setters are asked to review the questions, bearing in mind the standard that a competent GP trainee should achieve.

In summary, the aim of standard setting is to improve the fairness and validity of the examination process and to set levels of competence for success in the examination. It is important to emphasise that the use of these methods is independent of any external factors.

FIGURE 1 | **The blueprinting process**

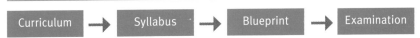

Curriculum ➡ Syllabus ➡ Blueprint ➡ Examination

The question formats' educational and evaluative benefits

The old-style DRCOG placed undue emphasis on a single style of response and subject matter: that of basic medical or clinical knowledge. While this has a place, and will continue to do so, the non-oral OSCE stations and MCQs in particular, tended to test similar material. The OSCE had its positive elements. The relatively realistic role-play stations were valued, although these were limited in number, and more sophisticated and testing versions appeared throughout the remainder of the GP training and assessment. Essentially, however, the OSCE was a poor discriminator compared with the MCQ paper. Bearing in mind that the MCQ paper in the new examination should improve in validity and reliability with the addition of other questions formats, and considering that the length of the old examination was excessive, a reduction in examination time was also justified.

All three formats of the new examination (EMQ, SBA and MCQ) can be computer marked, which is of great practical advantage in replacing short open-answer questions. Computer marking is more accurate, more reliable and faster.

Moreover, the combination of the three question formats has sound, 'added value' educational and evaluative benefits. That is to say, they should drive effective learning and improve discrimination in placing the correct candidates on either side of the pass or fail boundary. Multiple indicators tend to increase an examination's validity, which is why the new examination uses a combination of all three question formats EMQ, SBA and MCQ. The mix of formats should ensure that candidates will need good and rounded study to pass, since rote learning without understanding is a potential pitfall of the learning and assessment process.

MCQs remain a valid part of the examination due to their thorough testing of cognitive (or factual) knowledge. Research demonstrates unequivocally that such knowledge is the single best determinant of expertise in a subject. The weaknesses of MCQs are that they predominantly test recall and some candidates answer correctly by a process of elimination rather than through actual knowledge. The College has been carefully trying to mitigate these weaknesses in its papers as far as is possible. For example, questions that test only obscure or isolated facts are avoided. This follows a large review of the format that clearly identified these as overly examined. Another pitfall of true or false MCQs is that a 'test-wise' candidate might guess correctly too often and gain a 'false' pass.

EMQs can probe certain areas, including some that are vital to clinical practice, such as management and the application of medical knowledge, far more effectively than other question formats. Most EMQs will define their clinical relevance quickly, which is not easy to accomplish with the MCQ format. They can also interrogate a candidate's understanding of the relationship between facts. Compared with true or false MCQs, the guessing of answers is more difficult and more complex understanding is tested. Close comparison in trials to all the other question formats demonstrates that EMQs can examine clinical problem solving particularly well. Modern psychometric methods indicate that the reliability of EMQ papers is generally very good. Moreover, a recent literature review of question formats in medical examinations concluded that 'there is a wealth of evidence that EMQs are the fairest format'. In that EMQs frequently use realistic clinical scenarios, they are a moderately more authentic sort of test, although this is secondary for the College compared to the validity and reliability they will add. EMQs require good clinical knowledge and its application across the broad range of obstetric and gynaecological practice. Within this, the essential domains of management, diagnosis and investigation will be the most frequently tested. An approach requiring good clinical reasoning skills will also be required.

The examination

The DRCOG examination is run twice a year, in April and October. The examination consists of two papers each lasting 90 minutes. There is a short break of approximately 15 minutes between the two papers. The approximate timetable (always check your College correspondence and/or the RCOG website) will be as follows:

09.45 Candidates are checked into the examination hall and the invigilator reads the examination instructions and clarifies any questions

10.00 Paper 1 begins, which consists of:
10 (× 3 stem) EMQs
18 single best answer (best-of-five) questions

11.30 Paper 1 ends

<small>BREAK</small>

11.45 Paper 2 begins, which consists of:
40 (× five-part) MCQs

13.15 Paper 2 ends

Mark weighting

The marks awarded to the three different question types vary. The EMQ and SBA questions will carry an extra 'weight' to reflect the increased difficulty of these questions and also the fact that they are not merely true or false and therefore do not carry a 50/50 chance of being answered correctly.

5 | Extended matching questions

EMQ structure

An EMQ is composed of three parts:
► a list of options
► a lead-in statement or paragraph (instructions)
► the items (questions).

The list of options will comprise ten or more words, phrases or numbers. Occasionally the option list will be shorter or longer. Possible list of options may include:
► diagnoses
► options for management
► pharmacological agents
► surgical procedures
► potential treatments.

Each question item or 'twig' will usually be a question based on a clinical scenario.

Writing effective EMQ format questions is not easy. The question authors have been guided to follow these writing guidelines to produce the bank of new questions:
► As far as reasonably possible the list of options is made homogeneous and widely different options are avoided.
► Vagueness is avoided. It is important that the candidate has a clear concept of exactly what is required at their first or second reading of the question.
► Each option is kept as short as possible and the use of verbs is avoided. However, as they are generally clinical scenarios, the items are often reasonably long.
► Lead-in statements are designed to link the items with the options and clarify the issues and task required for the candidate as much as possible.

What are the main differences between EMQs and the more familiar question formats? With the wider number of options available, it is obvious that the educated guess becomes a far less valuable technique than in the 50/50 case of the true or false MCQ. This does not mean that an educated guess is not sometimes appropriate for EMQs. The popular and renowned advice to trust the first answer you think of first is gaining ever more support. Essentially, for the EMQs, knowledge and clinical judgement are the vital requirements and any guessing needs to be judicious.

Answering EMQs

Candidates should find this technique useful in tackling EMQs:
1. Read the 'lead in' statement first.
2. Ask yourself the question: 'Do I really understand what the lead-in statement says?'
3. Consider each question one by one.
4. Develop the answer to the question in your mind.
5. Finally, select the correct answer from the list of options and enter your answer on the mark sheet.

Candidates are not advised to read through the list of options first. There is a small but live possibility of being wrongly cued by distractors among the options by doing this. The lead-in statement will generally be very clear as to the task required and should leave no room for ambiguity. Reading it carefully and understanding it will be the key to performing the task required in the correct manner and so answering the question accurately. Thus, for candidates with an appropriate standard of knowledge and experience, it will be a simple matter to answer the questions.

The DRCOG examination Paper 1 will contain ten EMQ questions. Each of these will consist of three twigs, all of which have to be answered by the candidate making a single selection from the answer option list provided. These will be marked at 3.5 marks per twig, giving a total mark of 105 out of the total 350 marks for the whole examination (30.0%). The EMQ questions will be derived from the entire syllabus.

We have prepared two EMQ papers, each containing ten questions, as in the examination, to aid your revision for the examination. The answers can be found in Chapter 15.

6 | EMQ paper one

Option list

A Atrophic vulvovaginitis	G Lichen simplex
B Endometriosis	H Vaginismus
C Recurrent candida infection	I Recurrent genital herpes
D Contact dermatitis	J Lichen planus
E Bartholin's cyst	K Lichen sclerosus
F Vulvodynia	

Each of the clinical scenarios below relates to a condition that may cause vulval problems in women. For each patient, choose the **single** most likely diagnosis from the list above. Each diagnosis may be used once, more than once or not at all.

Questions

1 ▷ A 21-year-old student presents with a 2-year history of vulval pain that is worse on intercourse. The pain with intercourse starts immediately with penetration. High vaginal swabs have been reported as negative. The vulva is normal with marked tenderness just below the urethral orifice.

2 ▷ A 60-year-old woman presents with chronic itching and soreness of the vulval area. She had her menopause at the age of 49 years and has never used hormone replacement therapy. On examination there is splitting of the vulval skin, atrophy of the vulva area with white areas distributed around the vulva and anus.

3 ▷ A 35-year-old nulliparous woman presents with recent history of vulval pain. She has complained of painful periods for many years and this has been controlled with the oral contraceptive pill and Tranexamic acid tablets. On examination she has a 3 cm swelling in posterior aspect of the left labium majus.

Option list

A 6-month course of gonadotrophin-releasing hormone (GnRH) agonist with add-back therapy
B Medroxyprogesterone acetate
C Danazol
D 12 month course of GnRH agonist
E Levonorgestrel-releasing intrauterine system
F Tranexamic acid
G Combined oral contraceptive pill
H Laparoscopic resection of endometriosis including endometrioma
I Total hysterectomy and bilateral oophorectomy
J Diagnostic laparoscopy
K Oral contraceptive pill and nonsteroidal anti-inflammatory drugs

Each of the clinical scenarios below relates to endometriosis or possible endometriosis. For each patient, choose the **single** most likely treatment from the list above. Each treatment may be used once, more than once or not at all.

Questions

4 ▷ A 29-year-old woman with known moderate endometriosis presents with an 18-month history of primary infertility. Your GP partner has excluded male factor problems and she appears to be ovulating. What is the appropriate investigation or management?

5 ▷ A 28-year-old woman with known mild endometriosis presents with painful heavy periods. She has two children. She had a termination of pregnancy last month following a contraceptive pill failure. What is the most appropriate management?

6 ▷ A 38-year-old woman with known extensive endometriosis presents with painful heavy periods. She has completed 6 years of unsuccessful fertility treatment. What is the most appropriate treatment?

Option list

A	1 in 100	G	1 in 400
B	1 in 600	H	1 in 45
C	1 in 4	I	1 in 2
D	1 in 20	J	1 in 2500
E	1 in 1000	K	1 in 8
F	1 in 250		

Each of the clinical scenarios below relates to antenatal risk. For each patient, choose the **single** most likely risk from the list above. Each risk may be used once, more than once or not at all.

Questions

7 ▷ A 45-year-old woman presents to antenatal clinic at 10 weeks of gestation with a singleton pregnancy. She has become pregnant after intracytoplasmic sperm injection treatment and the eggs were donated by her 39-year-old sister. She wants to know the risk of karyotypic abnormality in this pregnancy.

8 ▷ A 32-year-old woman presents to the antenatal clinic at 15 weeks of gestation. She is fit and well with no significant family history. An ultrasound scan at 11 weeks showed a singleton pregnancy with no obvious fetal anomaly. She requests serum screening for Down syndrome and asks at what risk she would be called back and advised that she was high risk and therefore should consider an amniocentesis.

9 ▷ A 26-year-old woman presents to the antenatal clinic at 12 weeks of gestation with a twin pregnancy. She and her partner are known to have sickle cell trait. What is the risk to each twin of sickle cell disease?

Option list

A Antepartum haemorrhage
  of uncertain cause
B Placental abruption
C In-utero fetal death
D Placenta praevia
E Threatened preterm labour

F Severe pre-eclampsia
G Vasa praevia
H Urinary tract infection
I HELLP syndrome
J Reflux oesophagitis
K Appendicitis

Each of the clinical scenarios below relates to patients with bleeding and/or pain in pregnancy. For each patient choose the **single** most likely diagnosis from the list above. Each diagnosis may be used once, more than once or not at all.

Questions

10 ▷ An Afro-Caribbean woman in her third pregnancy presents with a sudden onset of painless vaginal bleeding at 33 weeks of gestation. Her previous deliveries were by emergency caesarean section.

11 ▷ An 18-year-old primigravida at 28 weeks of gestation presents with epigastric pain, complaining of feeling generally unwell with absent fetal movements. On examination she is afebrile and the symphysis-fundal height is small for dates. Investigations include a normal white cell count, platelet count of 145, normal urea and electrolytes and abnormal liver function tests with a raised AST (aspartame aminotransferase) level.

12 ▷ A 32-year-old woman in her first pregnancy presents at 30 weeks of gestation with colicky lower abdominal pain, mainly to the right side, of 3 hours' duration. On examination, she is apyrexial, she has no vaginal bleeding but has a vaginal discharge consistent with bacterial vaginosis. There is generalised abdominal tenderness. A cardiotocograph is reassuring.

Option list

A Chorion villus sampling at 11 weeks of gestation
B Amniocentesis
C Detailed ultrasound scan at 20 weeks of gestation
D Serum screening with human chorionic gonadotrophin/alpha fetoprotein/estriol levels
E Nuchal translucency scan
F Chorionic villus sampling at 8 weeks of gestation
G Third-trimester growth scan
H Karyotype both parents for balanced (Robertsonian) translocation
I Combined nuchal translucency scan and serum screening
J Cordocentesis for karyotype
K Serum alpha-fetoprotein level

The clinical scenarios below relate to pre-natal diagnosis. For each patient, select the **single** most appropriate investigation. Each option may be used more than once or not at all.

Questions

13 ▷ The wife of your business manager comes to see you at 10 weeks of gestation because she has conceived unexpectedly many years after the birth of her last child. This is her fifth pregnancy, they have three teenage children and she had a termination of pregnancy in similar circumstances last year. She is 40 years of age and wants a diagnostic test to exclude Down syndrome as soon as possible.

14 ▷ A 25-year-old woman presents at 16 weeks of gestation. She has a healthy 4-year-old child and last year had a termination of pregnancy at 14 weeks, following a diagnosis of anencephaly. She wishes to have the most sensitive test in this current pregnancy to exclude anencephaly and related conditions.

15 ▷ A couple present at 6 weeks of gestation in their first pregnancy. They know that they are both carriers of cystic fibrosis. They request prenatal diagnosis.

Option list

A   Pregnancy can normalise hypothyroidism and therefore the dose of thyroxine replacement should only be increased in early pregnancy after checking thyroid function tests

B   Women receiving thyroxine should continue on the same dose until seen in a consultant-led clinic

C   Women receiving thyroxine should increase the daily dose by up to 50% as soon as they have a positive pregnancy

D   Adequate treatment with thyroxine in pregnancy limits the risks of miscarriage, late pregnancy complications and neurodevelopmental delay in the offspring

E   Any under-treatment of hypothyroidism in pregnancy is associated with clear neurodevelopmental delay in the offspring

F   Women receiving thyroxine should increase the daily dose by up to 30% as soon as they have a positive pregnancy test

G   The daily dose of thyroxine should be decreased to preconception levels in the first 4 weeks postpartum

H   Women with treated hypothyroidism should increase the daily dose of thyroxine prepregnancy

I   The main cause of hypothyroidism in the UK is iodine deficiency and she should therefore increase the amount of iodine in her diet

J   Postpartum, the thyroid function tests should be repeated every 6 months with a view to reducing thyroxine replacement

Each of the clinical scenarios below relates to women with hypothyroidism and pregnancy. For each woman, choose the **single** most likely statement that the GP would be heard to say from the list above. Each statement may be used once, more than once or not at all.

Questions

16 ▷ A 22-year-old woman with treated hypothyroidism presents for prepregnancy counselling. She wishes to know the implications of her condition upon the pregnancy and the fetus.

17 ▷ The woman returns to the surgery 4 months later at 9 weeks of gestation. She wishes to know how she should manage her thyroxine replacement therapy in pregnancy.

18 ▷ The woman returns to see you 4 days following the successful delivery of a daughter at term, with mastitis. She continues to take the predelivery dose of thyroxine. She takes the opportunity to ask how she should manage her thyroxine replacement now that she has delivered.

Option list

A Recurrent urinary tract infection
B Endometriosis
C Anovulatory cycles
D Juvenile type Granulosa cell ovarian tumour
E Fibroids
F Pregnancy
G Von Willebrand's disease
H Polycystic ovary syndrome
I Anorexia nervosa
J Haematocolpos
K Chronic pelvic inflammatory disease

Each of the clinical scenarios below relates to adolescent women with bleeding and/or pain. For each patient choose the **single** most likely diagnosis from the list above. Each diagnosis may be used once, more than once or not at all.

Questions

19 ▷ A 16-year-old woman presents heavy irregular bleeding since a menarche 12 months ago. She has a body mass index of 20 and is also concerned about excess hair growth and facial 'spots'. She is accompanied by her mother, who has no history of gynaecological problems. On examination, there is no evidence of hirsutism or acne.

20 ▷ A 16-year-old African woman presents with several episodes of lower abdominal pain associated with dysuria over the past few months. The history is relevant for female genital mutilation at the age of 11 years. She has regular painless light periods. Repeated urine samples have shown no evidence of infection.

21 ▷ A 15-year-old schoolgirl presents with cyclical pelvic pain. She has not yet started menstruating. Examination showed an appropriate Tanner stage of development.

Option list

A Levonorgestrel-releasing intrauterine system
B Combined oral contraceptive pill
C Progesterone-only pill
D GnRH agonist with add-back therapy
E Dianette®
F Depo-Provera®
G Clomifene citrate
H Cyclical medroxyprogesterone acetate
I Norethisterone from day 5 to day 26 of each cycle
J Norethisterone from day 12 to day 26 of each cycle
K Oral mefenamic acid or tranexamic acid

Each of the clinical scenarios below relates to women with irregular, non-cyclical bleeding in the absence of pathology. For each patient choose the **single** most appropriate treatment from the list above. Each treatment may be used once, more than once or not at all.

Questions

22 ▷ A 22-year-old nulliparous lesbian woman requests treatment for menorrhagia and primary dysmenorrhoea. She also has troublesome mid-cycle bleeding. She has not had treatment for these conditions in the past.

23 ▷ A 35-year-old woman presents with a 2-year history of irregular bleeding, obesity and hirsutism. She has not used contraception since stopping Yasmin® (Schering Health) 2 years ago and is keen to be pregnant.

24 ▷ A 49-year-old woman presents with chaotic perimenopausal bleeding and menorrhagia. She weighs 92 kg, is a non-smoker and has a normal blood pressure. She has no other climacteric symptoms.

Option list

A Angiotensin-converting
   enzyme inhibitors
B Anticonvulsants
C Fluoxetine
D Cimetidine
E Tricyclic antidepressants

F Metoclopramide
G Metronidazole
H Propranolol
I Statins
J Tetracycline
K Warfarin

Each of the clinical scenarios below relates to drug treatment associated with fetal or neonatal anomaly. For each case, choose the **single** most appropriate drug treatment from the list above. Each treatment may be used once, more than once or not at all.

Questions

25 ▷ Oligohydramnios in the third trimester of pregnancy and renal tract malformation.

26 ▷ Defective ossification with mid-face hypoplasia, saddle nose and cardiac abnormalities in the neonate.

27 ▷ Neural tube defect detected on 20-week fetal anomaly scan.

Option list

A Alcohol	F Ecstasy
B Amphetamines	G Heroin
C Benzodiazepines	H Solvents
D Cannabis	I Methadone
E Cocaine	J Tobacco

Each of the clinical scenarios below relates to drug misuse in pregnancy. For each case, choose the **single** most appropriate drug misuse from the list above. Each treatment may be used once, more than once or not at all.

Questions

28 ▷ Placental abruption associated with fetal death in the third trimester.

29 ▷ Hypertension with no proteinuria and a normal full blood count at repeated visits in the second trimester of pregnancy.

30 ▷ Delivery of a growth-restricted fetus with microcephaly at term. The neonatal face is characterised by short palpebral fissures (eye openings) and a thin upper lip. The baby appears to have increased tone.

7 | EMQ paper two

Options list

A Atonic bladder
B Diabetes mellitus
C Diabetes insipidus
D Vesicovaginal fistula
E Overflow incontinence

F Stress incontinence
G Urge incontinence
H Urine tract infection
I Mixed urinary incontinence
J Urge syndrome

Each of the clinical scenarios below relates to lower urinary tract problems. For each case, choose the **single** most appropriate diagnosis from the list above. Each diagnosis may be used once, more than once or not at all.

Question

1 ▷ A 38-year-old multiparous woman presents with a long history of deteriorating incontinence. She has problems with urine loss and wetting herself with coughing sneezing or certain exercises and also describes 'door-key incontinence' when she cannot get to the toilet quickly enough.

2 ▷ A 62-year-old woman presents with a long history of wanting to go to the toilet frequently. She has a 2-year history of type 2 diabetes and is diet controlled. She passes small quantities of urine 10–20 times daily and has to get up 4–6 times per night. She has no urinary incontinence.

3 ▷ A 46-year-old woman presents with constant urinary leakage since the time of a total abdominal hysterectomy 3 weeks ago. She requires constant protection, at day and night.

Option list

A Acute myeloid leukaemia
B Aplastic anaemia
C Folic acid deficiency
D Thalassaemia
E G-6-PD (glucose-6-phosphate dehydrogenase) deficiency
F Physiological
G Sickle cell disease
H Iron deficiency
I Vitamin B12 deficiency
J Haemolytic anaemia

Each of the clinical scenarios below relates to anaemia in pregnancy. For each case, choose the **single** most appropriate diagnosis from the list above. Each diagnosis may be used once, more than once or not at all.

Questions

4 ▷ A haemoglobin of 10.8 g/dl is noted in a 28-year-old woman of Pakistani origin of 24 weeks of gestation. She is in her third pregnancy and states that she has poor intake of fresh vegetables. The mean corpuscular volume (MCV) is 95 fl.

5 ▷ A 28-year-old white woman with a gluten sensitive enteropathy is noted to have a haemoglobin of 8 g/dl and an MCV of 105 fl on booking bloods taken at 11 weeks of gestation.

6 ▷ A 25-year-old Cypriot woman attends clinic and tells you that she has just found out that she is pregnant. Blood results reveal a haemoglobin of 10.8 g/dl, a MCV of 72 fl, a mean corpuscular haemoglobin (MCH) of 25 pg/cell (27–32 pg/cell) and normal mean corpuscular haemoglobin concentration (MCHC) 330 g/l (320–350 g/l).

Option list

A Advise to stop breastfeeding and treat with appropriate emollient and topical steroid
B Ultraviolet B
C Emollients and -potent topical steroids applied after breastfeeding
D Ciclosporin

E Azothioprine
F Topical tacrolimus
G Methotrexate
H Psoralen and ultraviolet A treatment (PUVA)
I Oral steroids
J Emollients and mild-to-moderate topical steroids applied after breastfeeding

Each of the clinical scenarios below relates to treatments for eczema. For each case, choose the **single** most appropriate treatment from the list above. Each treatment may be used once, more than once or not at all.

Questions

7 ▷ A 28-year-old breastfeeding mother presents 4 weeks postpartum with eczema of the nipple and areola.

8 ▷ A woman on this effective treatment for moderate to severe eczema should be advised that it is contraindicated in pregnancy and breastfeeding and should be stopped 3 months prior to conception.

9 ▷ A woman on this treatment in early pregnancy should be advised that it is associated with cleft lip and palate in mice but appears to be safe in humans.

Option list

A Placental abruption secondary to antiphospholipid syndrome
B Twin–twin transfusion syndrome in a multiple pregnancy
C Placental abruption
D Appendicitis
E Urinary tract infection
F Acute polyhydramnios
G Degenerating fibroid
H Premature rupture of membranes with chorioamnionitis
I Cervical weakness resulting in threatened preterm labour
J Premature rupture of membranes

Each of the clinical scenarios below relates to pain in pregnancy. For each case, choose the **single** most appropriate diagnosis from the list above. Each diagnosis may be used once, more than once or not at all.

Questions

10 ▷ A 24-year-old woman in her first pregnancy presents at 28 weeks with uterine contractions and pain, with a temperature and flu-like symptoms. She reports a 3-day history of leakage of clear fluid vaginally that has now become offensive. In the past, she has had a cone biopsy for treatment of persistent cervical intraepithelial neoplasia I.

11 ▷ A 31-year-old woman in her first pregnancy at 30 weeks with dichorionic, diamniotic twins presents with a history of uterine contractions having noticed her abdomen bloat over the previous 48 hours. The 20-week anomaly scan suggested that one of the twins had a tracheoesophageal fistula. On examination, the uterus is large for dates and tense. Fetal parts are difficult to palpate.

12 ▷ A 32-year-old Nigerian woman presents at 24 weeks of gestation with severe colicky abdominal pain. She has had two previous pregnancies. The first was complicated by a postpartum deep vein thrombosis and the second resulted in a miscarriage at 20 weeks of gestation. She has just arrived in the UK and when seen in the antenatal clinic last week for the first time was noted to have fetal growth restriction on ultrasound scan in addition to a 6-cm fundal fibroid.

Option list

A Advise that she should continue statin use until seen by obstetrician at booking clinic
B Take periconceptual folic acid 0.4 mg/day
C Aim for blood glucose levels of 4.5–6.5 mmol/l
D Discontinue ACE inhibitor in early pregnancy
E Advice that advantage of ACE inhibitor outweighs risk throughout pregnancy

F Advice to maintain good blood sugar control as it will reduce the risk of miscarriage
G Take preconceptual folic acid 5mg/day until positive pregnancy test and seek medical advice as early as possible in pregnancy
H Seek medical advice as early as possible in pregnancy
I Check for retinopathy
J Change ACE inhibitor to alternative anti-hypertensive treatment
K Aim for blood sugar levels of 3.0–5.5 mmol/l

Each of the clinical scenarios below relates to insulin–dependent diabetes and pregnancy. For each case, choose the **single** most appropriate management from the list above. Each management may be used once, more than once or not at all.

Questions

13 ▷ A 31-year-old woman with a 25-year history of insulin-dependent diabetes presents at 5 weeks of gestation. She has had excellent blood sugar control and is on no therapy except insulin. Her blood sugar control has been erratic for the past 2 weeks because of nausea.

14 ▷ A 24-year-old woman requests advice regarding her ACE inhibitor therapy. She is about to stop her contraception in order to conceive and is worried about the associated risk to the fetus.

15 ▷ A 19-year-old woman with an 18-month history of very well controlled diabetes seeks your preconception advice.

Option list

A Repeat serum CA125 and pelvic ultrasound scan
B Urgent referral to gynaecological oncology team
C Routine referral to gynaecologist
D Urgent referral to gynaecologist
E Routine referral to gynaecological oncologist
F Reassure

G Repeat pelvic ultrasound scan at beginning of next cycle
H Repeat serum CA125
I Repeat pelvic ultrasound scan
J Advice that she requires hysterectomy and refer to appropriate gynaecologist

Each of the clinical scenarios below relates to incidental ovarian cysts found on ultrasound scan. For each case, choose the **single** most appropriate management from the list above. Each management may be used once, more than once or not at all.

Questions

16 ▷ A 55-year-old woman with left iliac fossa pain is found to have a 4-cm simple right ovarian cyst. A serum CA125 sample is measured at 40 u/ml.

17 ▷ A 33-year-old woman with menorrhagia is found to have a 5-cm right ovarian cyst with a single septation. The serum CA125 level is 12 u/ml.

18 ▷ A 48-year-old woman with nausea and bloating is found to have a complex multicystic right ovarian mass of 10 cm with a small amount of ascites.

Option list

A Aim for hospital-based vaginal delivery
B Induction of labour in the next few days
C Induction of labour at 38 weeks of gestation
D Elective caesarean section at 38 weeks of gestation
E Elective caesarean section at 39 weeks of gestation
F Aim for vaginal delivery with epidural for pain relief
G Aim for home birth
H Induction of labour at 41 weeks of gestation
I External cephalic version at 35 weeks of gestation
J External cephalic version at 37 weeks of gestation

Each of the clinical scenarios below relates to antenatal care where advice is required regarding the presentation or mode of delivery. For each case, choose the **single** most appropriate management from the list above. Each management may be used once, more than once or not at all.

Questions

19 ▷ A 32-year-old woman in her second pregnancy presents at 34 weeks of gestation with a breech presentation. Her previous delivery was by emergency caesarean section.

20 ▷ A 22-year-old woman at 36 weeks in her first pregnancy requests delivery at home. She has had no obstetric problems but is known to have ruptured membranes for the past 8 hours.

21 ▷ A 19-year-old woman in her first pregnancy presents at 37 weeks of gestation with a diastolic BP of 100 mmHg and ++ proteinuria. A diagnosis of moderate pre-eclampsia is made. A cardiotocograph is normal but the symphysis–fundal height is less than expected.

Option list

A Trichomonas	F Herpes
B *Chlamydia trachomatis*	G Primary herpes
C Syphilis	H Cervicitis with human papillomavirus
D Gonococcus	I Bacterial vaginosis
E Candida	J Group B streptococcal infection

Each of the clinical scenarios below relates to genital tract infection. For each case, choose the **single** most appropriate diagnosis from the list above. Each diagnosis may be used once, more than once or not at all.

Questions

22 ▷ A sex worker presents with a vaginal discharge that she describes as 'greeny-yellow and frothy with a fishy smell'. Intercourse has been painful and she has soreness when passing urine.

23 ▷ A 24-year-old married woman presents with a 3-week history of an abnormal vaginal discharge with an unpleasant smell, especially after intercourse. She also has burning during urination and vulval itching.

24 ▷ An 18-year-old student presents with painful urination and an increasing amount of vaginal discharge. She also complains of a throat infection and has had a fever. She is using the combined oral contraceptive pill and had a withdrawal bleed 2 weeks ago.

Option list

A Hysteroscopy under general anaesthesia
B Hysteroscopy under local anaesthesia
C Endometrial biopsy and pelvic ultrasound
D Endometrial biopsy
E Cervical cytology and pelvic ultrasound scan
F Cervical cytology
G Transvaginal pelvic ultrasound scan
H Screen for genital tract infection
I Vulval biopsy
J Colposcopy

Each of the clinical scenarios below relates to gynaecological problems. For each case, choose the **single** most appropriate management from the list above. Each management may be used once, more than once or not at all.

Questions

25 ▷ A 31-year-old woman attends for repeat cervical cytology 6 months after a 'borderline' result. When reported this test is described as 'mild dyskaryosis'. She also complains of lower abdominal pain of 6 months' duration.

26 ▷ A nulliparous woman of 55 years of age presents with a single episode of heavy painful postmenopausal bleeding. She has never had cervical cytology because of a fear of internal examinations.

27 ▷ A 62-year-old woman presents with a single episode of painless bleeding. She also complains of a persistent pain in the left-lower abdomen. Her family history includes two sisters with ovarian cancer.

Option list

A Tamoxifen
B Raloxifene
C Estrogen-only hormone replacement
D Oral continuous combined hormone replacement therapy
E Combined oral contraceptive pill
F GnRH agonist
G GnRH agonist with estrogen add-back therapy
H Levonorgestrel-releasing intrauterine system (Mirena®, Schering Health)
I Anastrozole (Arimidex®, AstraZeneca)
J Tranexamic acid

Each of the clinical scenarios below relates to gynaecological treatments. For each case, choose the **single** most appropriate treatment from the list above. Each treatment may be used once, more than once or not at all.

Questions

28 ▷ This treatment option is associated with a 30–50% reduction in menstrual blood loss with typical adverse effects of 'feeling queasy' and leg cramps.

29 ▷ This aromatase inhibitor can be prescribed to postmenopausal women with estrogen-sensitive tumours. Adverse effects include nausea, flushes and sweats and lethargy. Thrombosis and loss of bone density are described.

30 ▷ This treatment option for climacteric symptoms is not associated with an increase in risk of breast cancer but may increase the risk of endometrial cancer if used in the long term.

8 | Single best answer (best of five) questions

'Single best answer' questions in the DRCOG examination have five possible answers (best of five), only one of which is correct. The other four answers should be reasonable to those with good knowledge but they are incorrect.

SBA (best of five) questions are increasingly used in Royal College and other UK postgraduate examinations. They are thought to mimic the way in which most doctors function in clinical situations: we see a patient, think of the possible diagnoses or management options and then decide on the most likely option from this list.

By adding SBA questions to the DRCOG examination it is believed that the examination will test decision making rather than merely the ability to recall facts. Because this tests a different skill from true or false MCQs, it is reasonable to assume that the validity of the DRCOG examination will be improved.

EXAMPLES

The SBA (best of five) questions will be in one of the two following forms:

Example 1

One of the following statements is **true**.

In pregnancy:

A ▷ Urine hCG levels are raised and this is used as the basis for urinary pregnancy tests.
B ▷ Early pregnancy vomiting is best treated with antiemetics.
C ▷ The symphysis–fundal height is an accurate screening test for intrauterine growth restriction.
D ▷ Maternal smoking has no deleterious effects on the fetus.

E ▷ An anomaly scan at approximately 20 weeks of gestation rarely fails to detect fetal abnormalities.

This type of SBA question presents you with five statements which are related by the stem 'In pregnancy' but the statements are otherwise unrelated. You are asked to select the statement that in your opinion is correct. Only one of the statements is correct. In this case, the correct answer is **A**.

Example 2

For the following clinical problem one of the following diagnoses is **correct**.

A 21-year-old primigravid woman presents at 7 weeks of gestation with vaginal bleeding and lower abdominal pain. A similar event the previous week was investigated in the early pregnancy unit. An ultrasound scan at that time showed an empty uterus and the plan was to repeat the scan in 2 weeks. The past medical history is significant for pelvic inflammatory disease with chlamydia and trichomonas.

A ▷ Threatened miscarriage.
B ▷ Ectopic pregnancy.
C ▷ Complete miscarriage.
D ▷ Incomplete miscarriage.
E ▷ Cervicitis.

This type of SBA question presents you with five diagnoses for the clinical problem. You are asked to select the diagnosis that in your opinion is correct. More than one of the diagnoses may be correct but you are expected to choose the diagnosis that is most likely to fit with the clinical history provided. In this case, the correct answer is **B**: ectopic pregnancy. The important fact that the patient has had an infection that may cause tubal disease makes this the correct answer, although all other answers could be correct. In other scenarios, the choice may be from a list of treatments, therapies or management options.

The DRCOG examination Paper 1 will contain 18 SBA questions. These will be marked at 2.5 marks per question, giving a total mark of 45 out of the total 350 marks for the whole examination (12.9%). The SBA questions will be derived from the entire syllabus.

We have prepared two SBA (best of five) papers, each containing 18 questions, to aid your revision for the examination. The answers can be found in Chapter 15.

9 | Single best answer paper one

1 ▶ One of the following statements is **true**.

In HIV infection:

A ▷ HIV screening should only be offered to pregnant women with risk factors for infection.

B ▷ Women found to be HIV positive on screening in pregnancy only require anti-retroviral therapy if the viral load is detectable.

C ▷ Commonly used anti-retroviral therapies are associated with a small risk of congenital anomalies when used in the first trimester.

D ▷ All pregnant women found to be HIV positive on screening in pregnancy should be delivered by caesarean section.

E ▷ A baby delivered to a woman with HIV infection should be initially treated with anti-retroviral therapy.

2 ▶ One of the following statements is **true**.

Regarding pre-eclampsia:

A ▷ Primigravid women should be screened more frequently than multigravidae.

B ▷ Hypertension is usually defined as greater than 140/100 mmHg.

C ▷ Weight gain of greater than 2 kg/week is significant.

D ▷ It does not occur in the absence of proteinuria.

E ▷ It is typically associated with symmetrical intrauterine fetal growth restriction.

3 ▶ One of the following statements is **true**.

A ▷ The stillbirth rate is defined as the number of infants born dead after 28 weeks of gestation per 1000 total births.

B ▷ Perinatal mortality includes all stillborn infants and those dying in the first 28 days of life.

C ▷ Maternal mortality rate is defined as the number of deaths per 1000 total births occurring during pregnancy and delivery.

D ▷ Early neonatal mortality is defined as all neonatal deaths in the first month of life.

E ▷ Infant mortality refers to all babies who die in the first 2 years of life.

4 ▶ One of the following statements is **true**.

Regarding the use of antibiotics:

A ▷ Prophylactic antibiotics should be given to all women undergoing emergency caesarean section but not elective caesarean section.

B ▷ Prophylactic antibiotics should be given to all women undergoing inpatient gynaecological procedures.

C ▷ Oral doxycycline for 14 days should be given to all women undergoing suction termination of pregnancy.

D ▷ Screening for infection should be performed prior to insertion of an intrauterine device or prophylactic antibiotics should be given.

E ▷ Metronidazole has an infrequent role to play in the treatment of gynaecological infections.

5 ▶ One of the following statements is **false**.

During the investigation of infertility:

A ▷ Ovulation can be confirmed using a midluteal phase progesterone level.

B ▷ A prolactin level is only required if the woman is anovulatory.

C ▷ Tubal patency is best confirmed by hysterosalpingogram in the majority of women.

D ▷ Metformin may have a role to play in the treatment of women with anovulation caused by polycystic ovary syndrome.

E ▷ Urine ovulation prediction kits are of value in treating couples with infertility of uncertain cause.

6 ▶ One of the following statements is **false**.

Regarding vaginal candidiasis:

A ▷ Predisposing factors include malignancy.
B ▷ Dysuria is a recognised symptom.
C ▷ Plaques or discharge may adhere to the inflamed vaginal walls.
D ▷ There is a characteristic fishy odour to the vaginal discharge.
E ▷ It is not necessary to treat the partner.

7 ▶ One of the following statements is **true**.

Rubella infection:

A ▷ Is rarely part of routine antenatal screening in the first trimester in primigravid women.
B ▷ Has an incubation period of 4 weeks.
C ▷ If acquired after the 16th week of pregnancy produces a congenital malformation in 20% of cases.
D ▷ Women found to be susceptible to rubella during prenatal screening should receive MMR vaccination before postnatal discharge.
E ▷ All pregnant women presenting with a vesicular rash compatible with a systemic viral infection should be investigated for rubella.

8 ▶ A 31-year-old woman with a history of three deep vein thromboses presents for prepregnancy advice. She is taking long-term warfarin and has no defined thrombophilia. She has never been pregnant. Which of the management options is **most** appropriate?

A ▷ Suggest that she continues on warfarin until she is pregnant. Inform her that she should return as soon as she has a positive pregnancy test.
B ▷ Suggest that she continues on warfarin until she is pregnant. Inform her that she should stop warfarin as soon as she has a positive pregnancy test.
C ▷ Suggest that she continues on warfarin until she is pregnant. Inform her that she should reduce the dose of warfarin as soon as she has a positive pregnancy test.

D ▷ Suggest that she switches from warfarin to heparin when she stops using contraception and continues on heparin in pregnancy.

E ▷ Suggest that she should not become pregnant.

9 ▶ One of the following statements is **true**.

Concerning premenstrual syndrome:

A ▷ GnRH agonists usually eliminate symptoms but treatment cannot be continued after 6 months.

B ▷ The combined oral contraceptive pill has not be shown to be effective in clinical trials.

C ▷ Antidepressants have no role in the treatment of this condition.

D ▷ It occasionally persists after the menopause.

E ▷ It always improves before or on the first day of menses.

10 ▶ One of the following statements is **false**.

Regarding bleeding in the third trimester:

A ▷ Placenta praevia is likely to present with unprovoked painless bleeding.

B ▷ Placental abruption may cause significant fetal compromise in the absence of heavy bleeding.

C ▷ Urgent referral to hospital is usually indicated.

D ▷ Requires administration of anti-D in rhesus-negative women whatever the cause.

E ▷ Requires investigation with an ultrasound scan in the majority of cases.

11 ▶ One of the following statements is **true**.

Absolute contraindications to prescribing the combined oral contraceptive include:

A ▷ Migraine in a 25-year-old woman.

B ▷ Recurrent benign cystic breast lesions.

C ▷ A body mass index of greater than 30.

D ▷ A past history of deep vein thrombosis.

E ▷ Cigarette smoking in women over 30 years of age.

12 ▶ One of the following statements is **false**.

Regarding the intrauterine contraceptive device (IUCD):

A ▷ A young women with a Nova T380 is using an appropriate IUCD.
B ▷ If an IUCD has not been expelled by 3 months it will not be expelled.
C ▷ A perimenopausal woman of 52 years using an IUCD for the past 8 years should not be advised to have the device changed.
D ▷ Actinomyces-like organisms found on cervical smear suggests that the device should be changed and antibiotics prescribed.
E ▷ Is contraindicated in women with HIV infection.

13 ▶ One of the following statements is **true**.

Regarding contraceptive methods:

A ▷ The pregnancy index (or Pearl index) for a 25-year-old woman taking a progestogen only pill is approximately 0.5/100 woman-years of use.
B ▷ Copper-bearing intrauterine devices are more effective in preventing pregnancy than injectables (Depo Provera®, Pharmacia).
C ▷ Non-smokers with no risk factors for myocardial infarction (MI) should be advised that there is a moderate increase in risk of MI with use of the combined pill.
D ▷ The pregnancy index (or Pearl index) for combined oral contraceptives is approximately 0.5/100 woman-years of use.
E ▷ Implanon® (Organon) is licensed for 5 years.

14 ▶ One of the following statements is **true**.

Relating to a girl under the age of 16 years:

A ▷ She is committing an offence if she has sexual intercourse.
B ▷ She can undergo termination of pregnancy without parental consent.
C ▷ If 'Lord Fraser competent', her decision to accept medical treatment can be overridden by a parent.
D ▷ The subdermal implant Implanon® (Organon) is not licensed for use in this age group.

E ▷ The doctor can only prescribe oral contraception without parental consent if she is already sexually active and at risk of pregnancy.

15 ▶ One of the following diagnoses is **correct**.

A 19-year-old primigravid woman presents with epigastric pain and nausea at 33 weeks of gestation. Her blood pressure is 140/85 mmHg and she is unable to provide a urine sample. A full blood count sampled routinely last week showed a normal haemoglobin; the haematocrit was raised and the platelet count was 110. The symphysis-fundal height is 28 cm.

A ▷ Obstetric cholestasis.
B ▷ Reflux oesophagitis.
C ▷ Pre-eclampsia.
D ▷ Cholecystitis.
E ▷ Renal failure.

16 ▶ One of the following diagnoses is **correct**.

A 33-year-old woman presents with a 9-month history of secondary amenorrhoea following cessation of the oral contraceptive pill which she had been taking for 6 years without problem.

Blood investigations include:

LH/FSH	5.2/3.6 u/l
Prolactin	455 mg/l
Testosterone	2.9 nmol/l
Estrogen	93 pg/ml (normal range 20–400)
T4	23.4 (range 9.8–23.1 pmol/l) TSH 1.7 mu/l (0.35–5.50 mu/l)

A ▷ Premature menopause.
B ▷ Polycystic ovary syndrome.
C ▷ Hyperprolactinaemia.
D ▷ Hyperthyroidism.
E ▷ Post-pill amenorrhoea.

17 ▶ One of the following management options is **correct**.

A 51-year-old woman presents with mild climacteric symptoms. Her last period was 2 years ago. She has a body mass index of 21 and is a non-smoker. She requests treatment to prevent osteoporosis as her mother has just died following a hip fracture related to a trivial fall. A DXA scan has been done and it shows evidence of osteopenia.

A ▷ Life-style advice including diet and repeat the DXA scan in 2 years.
B ▷ Continuous combined hormone replacement therapy.
C ▷ Tibolone.
D ▷ A bisphosphonate.
E ▷ Oral calcium supplementation.

18 ▶ One of the following management options is most **appropriate**.

A 34-year-old woman presents with menorrhagia. She has two children, feels her family is complete and uses the progestogen-only pill for contraception. She has no intermenstrual or postcoital bleeding. She has a body mass index of 28 and is a cigarette smoker. She is willing to consider any options for the management of the menorrhagia.

A ▷ Mirena® (Schering Health) intrauterine system.
B ▷ Endometrial ablation.
C ▷ Combined oral contraceptive pill.
D ▷ Depo Provera® (Pharmacia).
E ▷ Tranexamic acid.

10 | Single best answer paper two

1 ► Which of the following diagnoses is most likely to be **correct**?

A 31-year-old woman with a body mass index of 36 presents with anxiety and acute dyspnoea 5 days after her first delivery. The delivery was complicated by a postpartum haemorrhage after an emergency caesarean section under general anaesthesia. She admits to being very depressed about her failure to breastfeed. Her only medication on discharge from hospital was oral iron supplementation. What is the likely diagnosis?

A ▷ Anaemia.
B ▷ Postoperative chest infection.
C ▷ Pulmonary embolism.
D ▷ Amniotic fluid embolism.
E ▷ Postnatal depression.

2 ► Which of the following is **correct**?

A 21-year-old woman with well-controlled epilepsy on sodium valproate 600 mg twice daily but presents with an unplanned pregnancy at 7 weeks of gestation. She has had no convulsions for 18 months until last week, when she had one convulsion. She has been taking oral contraceptives for 3 years.

A ▷ An alternative anticonvulsant should be used in place of sodium valproate.
B ▷ Interaction of sodium valproate with the oral contraceptive increases the risk of congenital anomaly in this pregnancy.
C ▷ The dose of sodium valproate should be increased or a second anticonvulsant agent introduced.
D ▷ There is an increased risk of a neural tube defect in her fetus.
E ▷ Termination of pregnancy should be offered.

3 ▶ Which of the following is **correct**?

The following drugs should not be prescribed for a breastfeeding mother?

A ▷ Anti-retroviral therapy.
B ▷ Erythromycin.
C ▷ Tetracycline.
D ▷ Methadone.
E ▷ Warfarin.

4 ▶ Which of the following is the most **appropriate** management?

A 14-year-old woman presents with issues regarding poor breast develop-ment and primary amenorrhoea. Otherwise, she has been quite well and has done well at school academically although is feeling self-conscious as she really has not developed compared with her classmates. On examination, she is of normal height, has a body mass index of 21.5, has poor secondary sexual characteristics with little breast development and no pubic or axil-lary hair.

A ▷ Refer to gynaecologist with interest in adolescent problems.
B ▷ Reassure that she is normal and that such developmental delay is common in your experience.
C ▷ Refer to paediatric consultant with interest in endocrine disorders.
D ▷ Take a hormone profile and karyotype. Review when results available.
E ▷ Reassure that developmental delay is within normal limits. Review in 6 months.

5 ▶ Which of the following would be **appropriate**?

A 34-year-old woman booked for community-led midwifery antenatal care presents at 28 weeks of gestation. She requests an elective caesarean section because she is terrified of 'giving birth naturally'.

A ▷ Ask community midwife to counsel and reassure.
B ▷ Inform that caesarean section is not an option as there is no indication.
C ▷ Refer to obstetrician for opinion.

D ▷ Recommend attendance at antenatal classes.

E ▷ Refer to obstetrician recommending a caesarean section.

6 ► Which of the following is **appropriate**?

A 39-year-old woman at eight weeks of gestation requests a diagnostic test for Down syndrome with the lowest possible risk of pregnancy loss.

A ▷ Serum screening at 15 weeks of gestation.

B ▷ Combined nuchal translucency test and first-trimester serum screening.

C ▷ Amniocentesis at 15 weeks of gestation.

D ▷ Chorion villus sampling at 11 weeks of gestation.

E ▷ Fetal anomaly scan at 20 weeks of gestation.

7 ► One of the following is **false**.

The following are used for endometrial ablation:

A ▷ Rollerball diathermy.

B ▷ Microwave ablation.

C ▷ Thermal balloon.

D ▷ Laser ablation.

E ▷ Implants to endometrium.

8 ► One of the following options is **most** appropriate.

A 55-year-old woman presents with symptoms of stress and urge urinary incontinence. You refer her to a physiotherapist for pelvic floor exercises but this is of limited success. On pelvic examination, she has a cystocele that descends to the level of the introitus.

A ▷ Anterior vaginal wall repair.

B ▷ Midurethral tape procedure.

C ▷ Colposuspension.

D ▷ Urodynamic bladder test prior to any intervention.

E ▷ Anterior vaginal wall repair with midurethral tape.

9 ▶ One of the following management options is **correct**.

A 27-year-old woman presents with a 5-month history of breakthrough bleeding on the combined oral contraceptive pill. She has never had cervical cytology. On examination, the cervix appears vascular and hypertrophied:

A ▷ Cervical cytology.

B ▷ Cervical cytology and screen for genital tract infection.

C ▷ Cervical cytology, screen for genital tract infection and refer for colposcopy.

D ▷ Screen for genital tract infection.

E ▷ Cervical cytology, screen for genital tract infection and refer to general gynaecologist.

10 ▶ One of the following is **false**.

The following indicate an increased risk of ovarian malignancy:

A ▷ A raised serum CA 125.

B ▷ An ovarian cyst with septations and solid components.

C ▷ A persistent ovarian cyst of greater than 3 cm diameter.

D ▷ A raised carcinoembryonic antigen (CEA).

E ▷ An ovarian cyst of greater than 5 cm in a postmenopausal woman.

11 ▶ One of the following is **incorrect**.

Regarding varicella:

A ▷ Most UK adults are nonimmune.

B ▷ Infection in the second half of pregnancy is not associated with an increased risk of congenital anomaly.

C ▷ Maternal infection within 4 weeks of the birth may result in severe life-threatening infection in the neonate.

D ▷ Infection in pregnancy is associated with a greater risk of complications in smokers.

E ▷ Immigrants from subtropical areas are less likely to be immune.

12 ▶ One of the following is **correct**.

Regarding miscarriage:

A ▷ The recommended medical term for pregnancy loss under 24 weeks is 'abortion'.

B ▷ When talking to women, it is more important to use accurate terms such as 'pregnancy failure', or 'incompetent cervix' even though they can contribute to negative self-perceptions and worsen any sense of failure.

C ▷ Modern monoclonal antibody based kits can detect hCG at 25 iu/l, a level reached 9 days after conception.

D ▷ Ultrasound assessment is unreliable in confirming the diagnosis of complete miscarriage.

E ▷ The majority of women attending an early pregnancy unit with a suspected ectopic pregnancy can be managed using urine-based hCG tests.

13 ▶ One of the following management options is **correct**.

A 31-year-old multiparous woman presents with 8 weeks of amenorrhoea and a positive pregnancy test. Her previous two pregnancies have been uneventful. She has hypothyroidism for which she has taken thyroxine 100 micrograms daily for the past 4 years. Her most recent thyroid function test taken 2 months ago revealed that she was euthyroid.

A ▷ Refer to high-risk antenatal clinic urgently.

B ▷ Decrease thyroxine requirements by 25–50 micrograms daily and refer to hospital antenatal clinic.

C ▷ Leave dose of thyroxine unchanged and refer to midwifery-led care.

D ▷ Refer to high-risk antenatal clinic routinely.

E ▷ Refer to endocrinology clinic routinely.

14 ▶ One of the following treatments is **most** appropriate.

A 25-year-old woman who is 12 weeks pregnant presents with continued vomiting and weight loss. On examination she has a pulse of 106 beats/

minute, appears dehydrated and urinalysis shows ketosis. You commence intravenous fluids and intramuscular antiemetics. Investigations reveal:

Free T4	25.5 pmol/l (range 9.8–23 pmol/l)
TSH	0.35 mu/l (range 0.35–5.0 mu/l)
TSH-R antibody	1.3 iu/l (normal < 2 iu/l)
Haematocrit	0.45
Haemoglobin	14.8 g/dl
Ultrasound scan	Live singleton fetus of size equal to dates.

A ▷ Vitamin B supplements and subcutaneous heparin.
B ▷ Carbimazole.
C ▷ Oral steroids, subcutaneous heparin.
D ▷ Vitamin B supplements.
E ▷ Carbimazole and propranolol.

15 ▶ One of these statements is **true**.

With respect to the injectable contraceptive preparation medroxyprogesterone acetate (DMPA):

A ▷ It is not associated with weight gain.
B ▷ It should be given by subcutaneous injection.
C ▷ By 1 year, 10% of women stop using DMPA because of irregular bleeding.
D ▷ It should be given every 15 weeks.
E ▷ Although conception can occur rapidly after an injection has been missed, patients should be warned that a delay in conception is not uncommon.

16 ▶ One of the following statements is **false**.

In the perimenopause:

A ▷ A copper intrauterine device inserted at the age of 44 years does not need to be changed for continued effective contraception.

B ▷ It is reasonable to assume that a woman of 47 years of age with a 24-month history of amenorrhoea and vasomotor symptoms is no longer fertile.

C ▷ A 52-year-old woman who does not wish to conceive should be advised to use contraception for a further 12 months after her menopause.

D ▷ An oral HRT preparation containing estradiol 2 mg taken once daily is not an effective contraceptive.

E ▷ Levonorgestrel-containing postcoital contraception is contraindicated because of the increased risk of ectopic pregnancy in older women.

17 ▶ One of the following statements is **true**.

Regarding hormone replacement therapy:

A ▷ Continuous combined estrogen and progestogen treatment should be recommended in the perimenopause if the woman wishes to avoid bleeding.

B ▷ The majority of currently available transdermal estrogen replacement patches should be changed every 3–4 days.

C ▷ Atrophic vaginitis in post menopausal women with a uterus can be treated with a topical estriol cream but requires addition of cyclical progestogens.

D ▷ Cyclical preparations contain 7 days of a progestogen per cycle.

E ▷ Transdermal estrogen patches may be applied to the abdomen, thorax, upper arms or thighs.

18 ▶ One of the following statements is **true**.

Regarding sexually transmitted diseases:

A ▷ Gonorrhoea commonly causes a profuse vaginal discharge.

B ▷ Genital warts are frequently a result of transmission from warts on the hand.

C ▷ Metronidazole is an effective oral treatment for vaginal thrush infection.

D ▷ Trichomoniasis infection in women is characterised by painful sexual activity without vaginal discharge.

E ▷ Genital *Chlamydia trachomatis* infection in the male may be asymptomatic in up to 50% of cases.

11 | Multiple choice questions

The DRCOG examination consists of two papers, the second of which is a 40-question MCQ paper with each question having five twigs to be answered **True** or **False** in 90 minutes.

There is no negative marking and so it advisable for candidates to answer all the questions, taking a guess at those of which they are unsure.

The paper is standard set and therefore has a variable pass mark, according to the difficulty of the paper and the standard setting principles and procedures described earlier (see Chapter 4).

The next two chapters contains practice papers. We have made every effort to ensure that these questions will be of a standard similar to that which you are likely to encounter in the examination. Once again, it is important to emphasise that the curriculum and syllabus will enable you to focus your learning on those subjects that are relevant to the UK-based GP. It is unlikely that you will be expected to have knowledge relevant to hospital-based practice unless the examiners consider it relevant, in which case it will be included in the curriculum and syllabus. For example, the examiners will not expect you to know the anatomy of the ureter but they may ask a question about the risk of injury to the ureter associated with hysterectomy, since a GP would be expected of to recognise or consider this complication of gynaecological surgery.

1 ▶ In ectopic pregnancy:

A ▷ The most common site is the tubal isthmus.
B ▷ The use of progestogen-only contraceptives is a recognised association.
C ▷ An 'intrauterine sac' will not be seen on pelvic ultrasound scan.
D ▷ A urinary pregnancy test will be positive in the vast majority of cases.
E ▷ A repeat ectopic pregnancy occurs in approximately 12% of cases.

2 ▶ The following statements regarding the investigation of hirsutism are correct:

A ▷ A serum testosterone of greater than 8 mmol/l is usual in polycystic ovary syndrome.
B ▷ A serum estradiol assay is indicated.
C ▷ Most cases are idiopathic.
D ▷ Transvaginal ultrasound scan is not indicated.
E ▷ Measurement of androstenedione and DHEAS may be helpful.

3 ▶ Concerning progestogen-only methods of contraception:

A ▷ Implanon® (Organon) delivers effective contraception for 5 years.
B ▷ Cerazette® (Organon) inhibits ovulation.
C ▷ The Mirena® (Schering Health) intrauterine system has a less than 10% discontinuation rate in the first year.
D ▷ They should be discontinued in users over the age of 50 years, even if the FSH level remains low.
E ▷ A Mirena® (Schering Health) intrauterine system cannot be used for endometrial protection as part of hormone replacement therapy.

4 ▶ The following statements regarding clomifene citrate are correct:

A ▷ There is a 10% risk of ovarian hyperstimulation syndrome.

B ▷ There is a 5% risk of multiple pregnancy.

C ▷ It should be used in conjunction with midluteal phase progesterone monitoring.

D ▷ It has little role in the management of couples with unexplained subfertility.

E ▷ In the majority of cases it should be prescribed for no longer than six cycles.

5 ▶ Female sterilisation:

A ▷ Fails in less than one in 500 cases.

B ▷ The failure rate is independent of the age at which the procedure is performed.

C ▷ Has a lower failure rate than the levonorgestrel-releasing intrauterine system.

D ▷ When the procedure fails, up to 50% of pregnancies occurring are ectopic.

E ▷ Has a lower failure rate than vasectomy.

6 ▶ Concerning women with chronic pelvic pain:

A ▷ Irritable bowel syndrome often has a cyclical presentation.

B ▷ Diagnostic laparoscopy is typically negative if the transvaginal ultrasound scan is normal.

C ▷ Pelvic inflammatory disease is a common cause.

D ▷ In women with a normal ultrasound scan, a trial of antibiotic therapy is often effective.

E ▷ Bladder disease is an important and not infrequent cause for pelvic pain.

7 ▶ Regarding substance misuse in pregnancy:

A ▷ Neonatal abstinence syndrome due to maternal benzodiazepine use is often more severe than that seen with other commonly used substances.

B ▷ opiate-dependent mothers should be discouraged from breastfeeding.

C ▷ Neonatal abstinence syndrome due to maternal methadone use typically presents after the first 24 hours.

D ▷ Marijuana users should be asked about frequency of use.

E ▷ All known substance misusers should be referred to a multidisciplinary antenatal clinic.

8 ▶ Overactive bladder:

A ▷ Is commonly referred to as an unstable bladder and can only be diagnosed on urodynamic studies.

B ▷ May be a symptom of multiple sclerosis.

C ▷ May arise in up to 10% of women after continence surgery with midurethral tape procedures.

D ▷ May be treated with bladder injections with botulinum toxin type A (Botox®, Allergan).

E ▷ Is best treated with oral or transdermal anticholinergic therapy.

9 ▶ Concerning surgical treatments of stress incontinence:

A ▷ Treatments include transvaginal and transobturator midurethral tape procedures.

B ▷ Midurethral tape procedures are now the first-line treatment for primary stress incontinence.

C ▷ Objective cure rates at 1 year are typically 75%.

D ▷ Periurethral injections are an option in some women.

E ▷ An anterior vaginal repair is not considered an option for the treatment of stress incontinence.

10 ▶ Risk factors for cervical cancer include:

A ▷ Cigarette smoking.
B ▷ Prolonged oral contraceptive use.
C ▷ Infection with *Chlamydia trachomatis*.
D ▷ Infection with HPV subtypes 12 and 6.
E ▷ A history of renal transplant.

11 ▶ The following statements regarding uterine fibroids are correct:

A ▷ Frequency of micturition may occur.
B ▷ Sarcomatous change should be considered if the uterine size increases rapidly.
C ▷ Embolisation of the uterine arteries is a treatment option in women who yet to complete their family.
D ▷ Subfertility may occur.
E ▷ Women of West African ethnicity are more likely to effected.

12 ▶ The following statements regarding cervical cytology and colposcopy are correct:

A ▷ Opportunistic screening should be offered to women presenting with suspected sexually transmitted infections.
B ▷ Mild dyskaryosis frequently reverts to normal within 6 months.
C ▷ Liquid-based cytology has a lower recall rate compared with traditional cervical screening techniques.
D ▷ Colposcopy is indicated if two consecutive cervical cytology results are reported as mild dyskaryosis.
E ▷ Colposcopy should not be performed in pregnant women.

13 ▶ Human papillomavirus:

A ▷ Is a small DNA virus.
B ▷ Plays an aetiological role in all common types of cervical cancer.
C ▷ May be detected on cervical cytology.
D ▷ Is more common in sexually active women under the age of 25 years.

E ▷ Can be successfully immunised against in sexually active young women.

14 ▶ Cervical ectopy:

A ▷ Is usually symptomatic.
B ▷ Is best treated in asymptomatic women.
C ▷ Does not occur on postmenopausal women.
D ▷ Causes an odourless vaginal discharge.
E ▷ May be associated with subfertility.

15 ▶ Clinical features typical of severe pre-eclampsia include:

A ▷ Occipital headache.
B ▷ Visual disturbance with central scotoma.
C ▷ Epigastric pain of hepatic origin.
D ▷ Retinal changes on ophthalmoscopy.
E ▷ An obligatory rise in blood pressure.

16 ▶ Complications which are characteristically associated with poorly-controlled insulin-dependent diabetes mellitus in pregnant women include:

A ▷ First-trimester miscarriage.
B ▷ Preterm delivery.
C ▷ Intrauterine growth restriction.
D ▷ A neonate at risk of convulsions.
E ▷ An increased risk of pre-eclampsia.

17 ▶ With regard to HIV infection in women:

A ▷ Cervical intraepithelial neoplasia is more common than in non-infected women.
B ▷ The combined oral contraceptive pill is contraindicated.
C ▷ Antiretroviral therapy should be commenced as soon as pregnancy is diagnosed.

D ▷ Vaginal delivery is not recommended if the viral load is undetectable.
E ▷ Intrauterine devices are relatively contraindicated.

18 ▶ The following should be avoided during pregnancy:

A ▷ MMR vaccine.
B ▷ Rubella vaccine.
C ▷ Tetanus vaccine.
D ▷ Varicella-zoster vaccine.
E ▷ Measles immunoglobulin.

19 ▶ Concerning the use of the following drugs in pregnancy and breast feeding:

A ▷ Sodium valproate use in pregnancy is associated with a risk of neural tube defects.
B ▷ ACE inhibitors cause significant fetal renal disease if used after the 16th week of pregnancy.
C ▷ Lamotrigine use in pregnancy is associated with an increased risk of oral clefting.
D ▷ Tricyclic antidepressants have a higher risk profile than serotonin reuptake inhibitors in pregnancy.
E ▷ Citalopram is present in high doses in breast milk.

20 ▶ Vaginal bleeding in the second trimester is associated with:

A ▷ Threatened preterm labour.
B ▷ Abdominal trauma.
C ▷ Placental abruption.
D ▷ Miscarriage.
E ▷ Essential hypertension.

21 ▶ Diagnostic amniocentesis at 16 weeks of gestation is associated with:

A ▷ An increased incidence of spontaneous miscarriage of approximately 0.5%.

B ▷ An increased incidence of talipes in the neonate.
C ▷ An increase incidence of breech presentation.
D ▷ An interval of 10 days before a result if using FISH techniques.
E ▷ A less accurate karyotype when compared with chorionic villus sampling.

22 ▶ Contraindications to the use of epidural analgesia in labour include:

A ▷ Maternal hypertension.
B ▷ Inherited thrombophilias.
C ▷ Backache after a previous labour with epidural use.
D ▷ Maternal cardiac disease.
E ▷ A body mass index greater than 40.

23 ▶ Puerperal pyrexia may be due to:

A ▷ Retained products of conception after a manual removal of placenta.
B ▷ Thrombophlebitis after an elective caesarean section.
C ▷ Mastitis in a breastfeeding mother.
D ▷ Epidural anaesthesia complicated by a dural tap.
E ▷ Group B streptococcus vaginal infection found on an incidental antenatal high vaginal swab.

24 ▶ Risk factors for deep vein thrombosis include:

A ▷ Progestogen-only contraceptives.
B ▷ Hyperemesis gravidarum with ketosis.
C ▷ Excessive blood loss at caesarean section.
D ▷ a body mass index greater than 35 in a combined oral contraceptive pill user.
E ▷ ovarian hyperstimulation syndrome.

25 ▶ The following statements concerning spontaneous twin pregnancy are correct:

A ▷ The perinatal mortality rate is higher for the second twin than the first twin.

B ▷ Fetal growth is best determined by ultrasound scan done at least every 4 weeks in the third trimester.

C ▷ Chorionicity is best determined by ultrasound scan at 20 weeks of gestation.

D ▷ Chorionicity is an important predictor of pregnancy outcome.

E ▷ The risk of delivery by caesarean section is no greater than that seen in singleton pregnancies.

26 ▶ Noncontraceptive benefits of the oral contraceptive pill in women over 40 years of age include:

A ▷ Regulation of menstruation.

B ▷ Fewer perimenopausal symptoms.

C ▷ A reduced risk of ovarian cysts.

D ▷ A reduced risk of osteopenia.

E ▷ A reduced risk of gall bladder disease.

27 ▶ Vaginal moniliasis:

A ▷ In characteristic form produces white plaques on the vaginal wall.

B ▷ Is defined as recurrent if it occurs more than more than three times per year.

C ▷ If recurrent in pregnancy, should be treated with oral fluconazole.

D ▷ If recurrent, typing and sensitivity testing is required.

E ▷ Is more common in young women who use long-term oral antibiotics for skin acne.

28 ▶ Lichen sclerosis of the vulva:

A ▷ Has a typical hour-glass distribution.

B ▷ Is characterised by thickened areas of white skin with loss of labial tissue.

C ▷ Should be biopsied to confirm the diagnosis as it is difficult to differentiate from vestibulitis.

D ▷ May be treated with topical steroids that should be initially used twice daily.

E ▷ Carries a lifetime risk of vulval cancer of approximately 5%.

29 ▶ Concerning alcohol and women's health:

A ▷ It increases the incidence of infertility.

B ▷ It is associated with an increased incidence of miscarriage.

C ▷ There is currently no consensus on the safe amount that can be consumed in pregnancy.

D ▷ If used in pregnancy, it increases the risk of learning disorders in offspring when tested at 7 years of age.

E ▷ Consumption during the first trimester carries the most risk.

30 ▶ Regarding prelabour rupture of membranes:

A ▷ If labour does not occur, induction of labour should be offered after 24 hours.

B ▷ Is associated with an increased incidence of operative delivery.

C ▷ It may be complicated by stillbirth.

D ▷ The mother should be treated with antibiotics.

E ▷ It can only be diagnosed by speculum examination.

31 ▶ Concerning the combined oral contraceptive pill:

A ▷ It is 98% effective in preventing teenage pregnancy.

B ▷ ED preparations contain 21 pills per pack.

C ▷ A monophasic pill is easier to use than a phasic pill if the woman wishes to avoid a withdrawal bleed.

D ▷ It reduces the lifetime risk of ovarian cancer.

E ▷ It should be discontinued in women who smoke at the age of 30 years.

32 ▶ Regarding postnatal mental health:

A ▷ Selective serotonin reuptake inhibitors (SSRIs) taken after 20 weeks of gestation cause no problems in the neonate.

B ▷ Tricyclic antidepressants have lower risks during pregnancy than other antidepressants.

C ▷ Fluoxetine is present in breast milk at relatively high levels.

D ▷ All antidepressants are associated with neonatal withdrawal syndrome that is usually mild and self-limiting.

E ▷ All SSRIs have the same risk profile in pregnancy.

33 ▶ With regard to the investigation of primary infertility:

A ▷ A first semen analysis reported as abnormal need not be repeated.

B ▷ In the presence of a normal pelvic ultrasound scan, a hysterosalp-ingogram is the first-line option for the assessment of tubal patency.

C ▷ A serum progestogen level done on day 21 of a 35-day cycle is sufficient to assess ovulation.

D ▷ A serum prolactin sample is best taken on day 3–5 of the cycle.

E ▷ Screening for genital tract infection, including *Chlamydia trachomatis*, is mandatory.

34 ▶ The following statements concerning rubella are correct:

A ▷ Congenital rubella syndrome is extremely rare after exposure to rubella vaccine in pregnancy.

B ▷ Primary maternal infection after the first trimester carries no risk to the fetus.

C ▷ Treatment with immunoglobulin reduces the risk of congenital abnormality.

D ▷ The risk of fetal anomaly after maternal infection in the first trimester is approximately 10%.

E ▷ MMR should be offered to nonimmune women immediately after delivery.

35 ▶ The following are associated with the polycystic ovary syndrome:

A ▷ Regular ovulatory cycles.
B ▷ Raised androgen levels, including testosterone.
C ▷ Hypertension.
D ▷ Increased insulin resistance.
E ▷ Bulky ovaries with multiple cysts up to 1 cm in size on ultrasound scan.

36 ▶ Proteinuric pregnancy-induced hypertension:

A ▷ Does not occur in multigravidae without a previous history of the condition.
B ▷ Is associated with fetal growth restriction.
C ▷ Is more common in twin pregnancies.
D ▷ Is commonly associated with hepatic dysfunction.
E ▷ Is associated with a raised platelet count.

37 ▶ When used to detect Down syndrome, nuchal translucency:

A ▷ Has a greater than 90% detection rate when combined with hCG and a pregnancy-associated plasma protein A test.
B ▷ May suggest the presence of a cardiac anomaly.
C ▷ May be combined with the presence or absence of the baby's nasal bone, to improve sensitivity.
D ▷ Is best measured at 11–13 +6 weeks.
E ▷ Is not an option in multiple pregnancy.

38 ▶ Regarding obstetric cholestasis:

A ▷ There is a risk of intrauterine fetal death.
B ▷ It is classically associated with generalised pruritus, pronounced on the palms and soles.
C ▷ Oral ursodeoxycholic acid does not have a role in its management.
D ▷ It can recur if the patient subsequently uses an estrogen-containing contraceptive pill.
E ▷ It can be diagnosed by measuring bile acid levels.

39 ▶ Regarding urodynamic studies:

A ▷ A pressure catheter is passed into the patient's rectum.
B ▷ A normal residual volume of urine is less than 30 ml.
C ▷ They may be complicated by a urinary tract infection.
D ▷ They should be performed prior to continence surgery.
E ▷ It is possible to differentiate between stress incontinence and urge incontinence.

40 ▶ Regarding hepatitis B infection diagnosed in pregnancy:

A ▷ The baby should be offered a vaccination programme that starts in the early neonatal period.
B ▷ Vaginal delivery increases the risk of transmission to the neonate.
C ▷ Breastfeeding should be discouraged.
D ▷ The mother should be referred to a hepatologist, infectious disease specialist or gastroenterologist after the pregnancy.
E ▷ The mother should be informed that the risk of transmission to her partner is small.

13 | MCQ paper two

1 ▶ Maternal smoking:

A ▷ Increases the risk of pre-eclampsia.
B ▷ Is associated with a decrease in cognitive function of the infant later in life.
C ▷ Cessation in pregnancy can be aided by use of transdermal nicotine replacement.
D ▷ Increases the risk of placental abruption.
E ▷ Is associated with a small increased risk of sudden infant death syndrome.

2 ▶ Periconceptual folic acid supplements of 5 mg daily are advisable when:

A ▷ The woman is using any anticonvulsant drug.
B ▷ The woman is taking long-term antibiotics for skin problems.
C ▷ The woman has insulin-dependent diabetes.
D ▷ Multiple pregnancy is more likely because of assisted reproductive techniques.
E ▷ There is a history of a neural tube defect.

3 ▷ The following statements regarding hirsutism are correct:

A ▷ It is defined as terminal hair growth in sites where only men normally develop such hair.
B ▷ Less than 50% of women consider themselves to be hirsute.
C ▷ The most common cause is polycystic ovary syndrome.
D ▷ Spironolactone may be used as a treatment.
E ▷ Topical eflornithine should be considered a first-line treatment.

4 ▶ With regard to the management of early pregnancy complications:

A ▷ Ectopic pregnancy can be managed by observation alone when hCG levels are falling.

B ▷ Serum hCG levels double every 7 days in the normal first trimester.

C ▷ Intramuscular methotrexate is a treatment option for a confirmed unruptured ectopic pregnancy.

D ▷ Fetal heart pulsation should always be seen when the crown rump length is equivalent to 7 weeks of gestation.

E ▷ An intrauterine gestation sac can normally be seen on a transvaginal ultrasound scan at 6 weeks of gestation.

5 ▶ Ultrasonography at 20 weeks of gestation allows determination of:

A ▷ The presence of Down syndrome in most cases.

B ▷ Gestational age, to within 3 days.

C ▷ The majority of cardiac defects when present.

D ▷ Placenta praevia.

E ▷ The presence of neural tube defects in more than 99% of cases.

6 ▶ Regarding the cervical HPV vaccine:

A ▷ It is not clear to what extent older women with prior HPV exposure could be protected by vaccination.

B ▷ HPV prophylactic vaccination may not be 100% effective and will probably not protect against all HPV types.

C ▷ It is currently recommended that all girls aged 13–15 should be given the cannot prescribe it privately.

E ▷ It consists of a course of 2 injections.

7 ▶ The following may be safely prescribed to a breastfeeding mother:

A ▷ Tricyclic antidepressants.

B ▷ Warfarin sodium.

C ▷ Levothyroxine.

D ▷ Methadone.
E ▷ Lamotrigine.

8 ▶ Regarding Down syndrome:

A ▷ It is often hereditary.
B ▷ It usually occurs following the fertilisation of an egg with 24 chromosomes.
C ▷ If suspected at birth, it will be confirmed by blood karyotyping in the first 24 hours.
D ▷ It is associated with general hypertonicity.
E ▷ It is not an indication for selective termination of pregnancy in a twin pregnancy.

9 ▶ Vaginal prolapse:

A ▷ Can be treated successfully with pelvic floor exercises in younger women.
B ▷ Is best treated with a ring pessary in most women over 60 years.
C ▷ When treated by surgical repair has a successful outcome in 90% of cases.
D ▷ May be caused by habitual straining due to constipation.
E ▷ May rarely be caused by a pelvic tumour.

10 ▶ Vulval pain is associated with the following conditions:

A ▷ Herpes simplex type I.
B ▷ Vulval vestibulitis.
C ▷ Lichen sclerosus of the vulva.
D ▷ Paget's disease of the vulva.
E ▷ Lichen planus.

11 ▶ Acute retention of urine in the female is associated with:

A ▷ Perineal surgery.
B ▷ Multiple sclerosis.

C ▷ Continence procedures.
D ▷ Acute herpes genitalis.
E ▷ Epidural anaesthesia for vaginal deliveries.

12 ▶ The following statements regarding tuberculosis (TB) and pregnancy are correct:

A ▷ Intrauterine fetal infection is common.
B ▷ A mother with untreated TB will rarely infect their newborn child.
C ▷ Untreated disease can cause preterm delivery.
D ▷ Diagnosis should be by microscopic sputum examination and culture.
E ▷ BCG vaccination is contraindicated.

13 ▶ Recognised causes of placental abruption include:

A ▷ Iron deficiency anaemia.
B ▷ Cocaine use.
C ▷ Road traffic accidents.
D ▷ Pre-eclampsia.
E ▷ Cigarette smoking.

14 ▶ Regarding syphilis:

A ▷ It can be acquired by oral, anal or vaginal sex.
B ▷ If left untreated, it follows a pattern of four stages.
C ▷ The small painless ulcer of primary syphilis typically appears within 7 days of sex with the infected person.
D ▷ A condom does not significantly reduce the risk of acquiring the infection.
E ▷ The ulcer of primary syphilis usually last up to 6 weeks.

15 ▶ An initial abnormal semen analysis requires the following further measures:

A ▷ Information regarding current medication.
B ▷ A repeat semen analysis.

C ▷ The administration of multivitamins.

D ▷ Referral to an assisted reproduction unit.

E ▷ Information on, and discussion about the timing of specimen collection.

16 ▶ The following statements about prolonged pregnancy are correct:

A ▷ It is defined as greater than 42 completed weeks of pregnancy.

B ▷ It is associated with an increased risk of caesarean section.

C ▷ Induction of labour should be offered after 41 completed weeks.

D ▷ Cervical sweeping is recommended prior to formal induction of labour.

E ▷ The risk of stillbirth is double that seen at 37 weeks of gestation.

17 ▶ Recognised aetiological factors in spontaneous miscarriage in the first trimester of pregnancy include:

A ▷ Congenital abnormalities of the uterus.

B ▷ Impaired glucose tolerance.

C ▷ Bacterial vaginosis.

D ▷ Previous loop diathermy excision for treatment of cervical intraepithelial neoplasia.

E ▷ Colposcopic examination in pregnancy.

18 ▶ Regarding estrogen and progestogen hormone replacement therapy in postmenopausal women:

A ▷ The increased risk of breast cancer is approximately three extra cases per 1000 women per year of use.

B ▷ There is a debate as to the association with stroke and myocardial infarction.

C ▷ There is no reduction in the risk of colorectal cancer.

D ▷ The risk of hip fracture is reduced within the first 5 years of use.

E ▷ There is an increased risk of venous thromboembolic events.

19 ▶ Regarding termination of pregnancy:

A ▷ It is illegal after 20 weeks of gestation.
B ▷ It should always be covered by prophylactic antibiotics.
C ▷ A contraceptive IUCD can be fitted during the procedure.
D ▷ It is associated with an increased risk of subsequent subfertility.
E ▷ If the contraceptive pill is to be used for contraception, it should be started 7 days after the procedure.

20 ▶ Vasectomy:

A ▷ Reversal within 5 years results in pregnancy in 90% of couples.
B ▷ Increases the risk of testicular tumours.
C ▷ Is effective after 4 weeks.
D ▷ Is associated with lower risk of post-procedure pregnancy than laparoscopic Filshie clip sterilisation in women.
E ▷ May be performed using a 'no scalpel technique'.

21 ▶ Regarding female genital mutilation:

A ▷ It is illegal in the UK, with possible imprisonment for anyone found guilty of performing the operation.
B ▷ Intentional reinfibulation following vaginal delivery is a reasonable option.
C ▷ It may result in prolonged labour.
D ▷ It is associated with retention of urine and recurrent urinary tract infections.
E ▷ It is associated with dysmenorrhoea.

22 ▶ The effectiveness of lactational amenorrhoea for contraception is reduced by:

A ▷ Reduced frequency of breastfeeding.
B ▷ The mother returning to work but still fully breastfeeding.
C ▷ Introducing supplements to the baby's diet.

D ▷ A baby of more than 6 months of age.

E ▷ Waiting for the first menstruation.

23 ▶ Regarding contraception and breastfeeding:

A ▷ The use of the combined oral contraceptive pill should be avoided for the first 12 weeks postpartum.

B ▷ The combined oral contraceptive pill can be used without restriction from 6 months postpartum.

C ▷ The use of the progestogen-only pill (POP) in the first 6 weeks postpartum has a small effect on breast milk volume.

D ▷ The use of the POP provides 99% efficacy.

E ▷ The use of the POP causes less problematic bleeding than in non-breastfeeding women.

24 ▶ The following may restrict the use of epidural analgesia in labour:

A ▷ A failed epidural in a previous labour.

B ▷ A heart murmur with a normal echocardiogram.

C ▷ Previous back surgery.

D ▷ Spina bifida occulta.

E ▷ Pustular psoriasis over the lumbar area.

25 ▶ With regard to menorrhagia:

A ▷ Tranexamic acid should be used as first-line treatment.

B ▷ Mirena® (Schering Health) is an effective treatment option in up to 85% of women.

C ▷ It requires investigation in women over 35 years.

D ▷ It may be treated by endometrial ablation in women who have yet to complete their family.

E ▷ It may be effectively treated with luteal phase progestogens.

26 ► Bilateral oophorectomy at the time of abdominal hysterectomy:

A ▷ Necessitates estrogen replacement therapy in women under 40 years of age.

B ▷ Is the usual treatment for endometrial carcinoma.

C ▷ Requires consent.

D ▷ Is appropriate in women over 50 years of age.

E ▷ Is recommended for pelvic endometriosis in a premenopausal woman.

27 ► The following are associated with dyspareunia:

A ▷ Trichomonas infection.

B ▷ Cervical intraepithelial neoplasia.

C ▷ Irritable bowel syndrome.

D ▷ Adenomyosis.

E ▷ Urinary tract infection.

28 ► Regarding the management of symphysis pubis pain in pregnancy:

A ▷ A specialist obstetric physiotherapy review is important.

B ▷ Acupuncture may have a role.

C ▷ Analgesia in the form of nonsteroidal anti-inflammatory drugs and paracetamol should be used.

D ▷ Induction of labour may be indicated.

E ▷ Spontaneous vaginal delivery is not recommended.

29 ► Regarding vulval lichen sclerosus:

A ▷ Water-based emollient creams are ineffective.

B ▷ Vulval biopsy is always advisable.

C ▷ The condition is self-limiting.

D ▷ The condition is associated with a 10% lifetime risk of vulval cancer.

E ▷ Topical steroid cream is the mainstay of treatment.

30 ▶ In maternal sickle cell disease:

A ▷ The risk of first-trimester miscarriage is increased.
B ▷ The incidence of pre-eclampsia is increased.
C ▷ The incidence of intrauterine growth restriction is increased.
D ▷ The male partner needs to be tested for haemoglobinopathies to allow accurate counselling.
E ▷ Antenatal diagnosis always requires chorion villus sampling.

31 ▶ Dysmenorrhoea typically:

A ▷ Responds to suppression of ovulation.
B ▷ Does not respond to prostaglandin synthetase inhibitors.
C ▷ Complicates the use of the intrauterine contraceptive device.
D ▷ Occurs in the presence of endometriosis.
E ▷ Responds to the combined oral contraceptive pill.

32 ▶ During the resuscitation of the neonate:

A ▷ The airway is best opened with the baby on its back with the head in a neutral position.
B ▷ If the baby is floppy, it may be necessary to apply 'chin lift' to effectively open the airway.
C ▷ The heart rate is best judged with a stethoscope.
D ▷ If the baby is not breathing adequately by about 30 seconds, you should give five inflation breathes.
E ▷ The ratio of compressions to inflations is four to one.

33 ▶ Recognised complications of first-trimester surgical termination of pregnancy include:

A ▷ Subsequent cervical weakness.
B ▷ A 5–8% incidence of long-term psychological sequelae.
C ▷ Rhesus isoimmunisation.
D ▷ Retained products of conception.
E ▷ Infertility.

34 ▶ The following statements about the climacteric are correct:

A ▷ An LH/FSH ratio is helpful in management of symptoms.
B ▷ The oral contraceptive pill is contraindicated.
C ▷ Bone density falls.
D ▷ Contraception is not required if the last menstrual period was 9 months ago in a 48-year-old woman.
E ▷ Typically lasts 12–24 months.

35 ▶ Regarding the use of oral emergency contraception:

A ▷ The failure rate is not dependent upon timing with unprotected sex.
B ▷ It consists of levonorgestrel 1500 mg and should be taken twice, 12 hours apart.
C ▷ It cannot be given twice in the same cycle.
D ▷ It is available over the counter.
E ▷ Nausea frequently occurs but vomiting only occurs in 1% of women.

36 ▶ Regarding uterine fibroids:

A ▷ When large, they cause infertility.
B ▷ They may be treated by embolisation if the woman is sure that her family is complete.
C ▷ They are associated with a 1–2% risk of sarcomatous change.
D ▷ They can be resected transcervically if they are subserous.
E ▷ When treated by uterine artery embolisation, a general anaesthetic is required.

37 ▶ Regarding anti-D prophylaxis given routinely usually at weeks 28 and 34 of pregnancy:

A ▷ Pregnant non-sensitised women who are RhD-negative should be strongly advised to have prophylaxis even if in a stable relationship with the father of the child and it is certain that the father is RhD-negative.
B ▷ Whoever is responsible for antenatal care should discuss prophylaxis

and explain the options available so that women can make an informed choice about treatment.

C ▷ Women who have opted to be sterilised after the birth of the baby may not require prophylaxis.

D ▷ There are National Institute for Health and Clinical Excellence guidelines regarding its use.

E ▷ It should be offered even if a potentially sensitising event occurred earlier in pregnancy that was covered by anti-D prophylaxis.

38 ▶ Regarding cord blood banking:

A ▷ The cord blood contains stem cells.

B ▷ The cord blood is usually collected as a routine and stored in public banks in the UK.

C ▷ A cord blood transplant can be use to treat many blood diseases and immune diseases.

D ▷ Cord blood can be frozen and stored for up to 10 years.

E ▷ It is inadvisable if delivery is premature.

39 ▶ Regarding preterm delivery:

A ▷ The risk is reduced by use of metronidazole in pregnancy.

B ▷ It is associated with preterm premature rupture of membranes.

C ▷ It is defined as delivery prior to 34 weeks of gestation.

D ▷ It is predictable if a detailed maternal and obstetric history is taken.

E ▷ It is an indication for consultant-led care in future pregnancies.

40 ▶ Regarding breech presentation at term:

A ▷ External cephalic version should be offered to all women unless a contraindication exists.

B ▷ The risk of fetal damage associated with external cephalic version is approximately one in 200.

C ▷ Vaginal delivery is associated with a high morbidity.

D ▷ It should rarely be missed on abdominal palpation.

E ▷ Investigation for associated conditions should always be performed.

14 | Ten tips for candidates

And finally, here are ten tips for DRCOG candidates:

1 ▶ Prepare for the examination well in advance. You will be better prepared for this examination if you have a breadth of clinical experience in women's health. Attend the clinics.

2 ▶ The whole of the syllabus must be covered by your reading and preparation.

3 ▶ Ensure that practice in answering all three of the question formats is included in your revision. There is ample evidence that increasing familiarity with the format improves performance.

4 ▶ Read the questions carefully, with particular reference to the lead-in statement and the items themselves in the EMQs and best-of-fives (SBAs).

5 ▶ For EMQs, attempt to generate the answer to the item first without reading the list of options.

6 ▶ For EMQs, once you have read the lead-in paragraph and read the item, choose the appropriate option from the list of options.

7 ▶ Be aware of 'distractors' in the EMQs and SBAs. These are options which could not possibly be correct.

8 ▶ If you do not understand a certain question then leave it for the time being, answer other questions and return to the difficult item at a later stage.

9 ▶ Make sure that you answer all the questions by the end of the examination. There is no negative marking.

10 ▶ Above all – control your stress levels – over-anxiety leads to excess adrenaline, with the risk of error in answering.

15 | Answers

EMQ paper one
(Chapter 6)

Question 1 = F
Question 2 = K
Question 3 = E
Question 4 = H
Question 5 = E
Question 6 = I
Question 7 = A
Question 8 = F
Question 9 = C
Question 10 = D
Question 11 = F
Question 12 = E
Question 13 = A
Question 14 = C
Question 15 = A
Question 16 = E
Question 17 = F
Question 18 = J
Question 19 = C
Question 20 = K
Question 21 = J
Question 22 = B
Question 23 = G
Question 24 = I
Question 25 = A
Question 26 = K
Question 27 = B
Question 28 = E
Question 29 = B
Question 30 = A

EMQ paper two
(Chapter 7)

Question 1 = I
Question 2 = J
Question 3 = D
Question 4 = F
Question 5 = C
Question 6 = D
Question 7 = J
Question 8 = G
Question 9 = I
Question 10 = H
Question 11 = F
Question 12 = A
Question 13 = C
Question 14 = D
Question 15 = G
Question 16 = A
Question 17 = G
Question 18 = B
Question 19 = E
Question 20 = B
Question 21 = B
Question 22 = A
Question 23 = I
Question 24 = D
Question 25 = J
Question 26 = A
Question 27 = C
Question 28 = J
Question 29 = I
Question 30 = C

Single best answer paper one (Chapter 9)

Question 1 = **E**
Question 2 = **A**
Question 3 = **B**
Question 4 = **D**
Question 5 = **E**
Question 6 = **D**
Question 7 = **D**
Question 8 = **A**
Question 9 = **B**
Question 10 = **D**
Question 11 = **D**
Question 12 = **E**
Question 13 = **D**
Question 14 = **B**
Question 15 = **C**
Question 16 = **B**
Question 17 = **D**
Question 18 = **A**

Single best answer paper two (Chapter 10)

Question 1 = **C**
Question 2 = **D**
Question 3 = **C**
Question 4 = **E**
Question 5 = **C**
Question 6 = **C**
Question 7 = **E**
Question 8 = **D**
Question 9 = **C**
Question 10 = **C**
Question 11 = **A**
Question 12 = **E**
Question 13 = **A**
Question 14 = **A**
Question 15 = **E**
Question 16 = **E**
Question 17 = **B**
Question 18 = **E**

Question 1	Question 6	Question 11
A = T	A = T	A = T
B = T	B = T	B = T
C = F	C = F	C = T
D = T	D = F	D = T
E = F	E = T	E = T

Question 2	Question 7	Question 12
A = F	A = T	A = F
B = F	B = F	B = T
C = T	C = T	C = T
D = F	D = T	D = T
E = T	E = T	E = F

Question 3	Question 8	Question 13
A = F	A = T	A = F
B = T	B = T	B = F
C = F	C = T	C = T
D = F	D = T	D = T
E = F	E = T	E = F

Question 4	Question 9	Question 14
A = F	A = T	A = F
B = F	B = T	B = F
C = T	C = F	C = T
D = F	D = T	D = F
E = T	E = T	E = F

Question 5	Question 10	Question 15
A = F	A = T	A = F
B = F	B = T	B = F
C = F	C = F	C = T
D = F	D = F	D = T
E = F	E = T	E = F

Question 16	Question 21	Question 26
A = F	A = T	A = T
B = T	B = T	B = T
C = T	C = F	C = T
D = T	D = F	D = T
E = T	E = F	E = F

Question 17	Question 22	Question 27
A = T	A = F	A = T
B = F	B = F	B = T
C = F	C = F	C = F
D = F	D = F	D = T
E = T	E = F	E = F

Question 18	Question 23	Question 28
A = T	A = T	A = T
B = T	B = T	B = T
C = F	C = T	C = F
D = T	D = T	D = T
E = F	E = F	E = F

Question 19	Question 24	Question 29
A = T	A = F	A = T
B = T	B = T	B = F
C = T	C = T	C = T
D = F	D = T	D = T
E = T	E = T	E = T

Question 20	Question 25	Question 30
A = T	A = T	A = T
B = T	B = T	B = T
C = T	C = F	C = T
D = T	D = T	D = F
E = F	E = F	E = F

Question 31
A = F
B = F
C = T
D = T
E = F

Question 36
A = F
B = T
C = T
D = F
E = F

Question 32
A = F
B = T
C = T
D = T
E = F

Question 37
A = F
B = T
C = T
D = T
E = F

Question 33
A = F
B = T
C = F
D = F
E = T

Question 38
A = T
B = T
C = F
D = T
E = T

Question 34
A = T
B = F
C = T
D = F
E = T

Question 39
A = T
B = F
C = T
D = T
E = T

Question 35
A = F
B = T
C = F
D = T
E = F

Question 40
A = T
B = F
C = F
D = F
E = F

Question 1
A = F
B = T
C = T
D = T
E = F

Question 2
A = F
B = F
C = T
D = F
E = T

Question 3
A = T
B = F
C = T
D = T
E = F

Question 4
A = F
B = F
C = T
D = T
E = T

Question 5
A = F
B = F
C = T
D = F
E = T

Question 6
A = T
B = T
C = F
D = T
E = F

Question 7
A = T
B = T
C = T
D = T
E = T

Question 8
A = F
B = F
C = T
D = F
E = F

Question 9
A = T
B = F
C = F
D = T
E = T

Question 10
A = T
B = T
C = T
D = T
E = T

Question 11
A = T
B = T
C = T
D = T
E = T

Question 12
A = F
B = F
C = T
D = T
E = T

Question 13
A = F
B = T
C = T
D = T
E = T

Question 14
A = T
B = T
C = F
D = F
E = T

Question 15
A = T
B = T
C = F
D = F
E = T

Question 16	Question 21	Question 26
A = T	A = T	A = T
B = T	B = F	B = T
C = T	C = T	C = T
D = T	D = T	D = T
E = F	E = T	E = T

Question 17	Question 22	Question 27
A = F	A = T	A = T
B = F	B = T	B = F
C = F	C = T	C = T
D = F	D = T	D = F
E = F	E = T	E = T

Question 18	Question 23	Question 28
A = F	A = F	A = T
B = T	B = T	B = T
C = F	C = F	C = F
D = T	D = T	D = T
E = T	E = T	E = F

Question 19	Question 24	Question 29
A = F	A = F	A = F
B = T	B = F	B = F
C = T	C = T	C = F
D = T	D = T	D = F
E = F	E = T	E = T

Question 20	Question 25	Question 30
A = F	A = T	A = T
B = F	B = F	B = T
C = F	C = F	C = T
D = T	D = F	D = T
E = T	E = F	E = F

Question 31
A = T
B = F
C = T
D = T
E = T

Question 36
A = T
B = T
C = F
D = F
E = F

Question 32
A = T
B = T
C = T
D = F
E = F

Question 37
A = F
B = T
C = T
D = T
E = T

Question 33
A = F
B = F
C = T
D = T
E = F

Question 38
A = T
B = F
C = T
D = F
E = T

Question 34
A = F
B = F
C = T
D = F
E = F

Question 39
A = F
B = T
C = F
D = F
E = T

Question 35
A = F
B = F
C = F
D = T
E = T

Question 40
A = T
B = F
C = F
D = F
E = T

Mock examinations answer sheets (blank)

Please feel free to photocopy these sheets
so that you can easily use and reuse them.

SBAs

Complete by fully filling in with pencil the lozenge corresponding to the **single** correct answer.

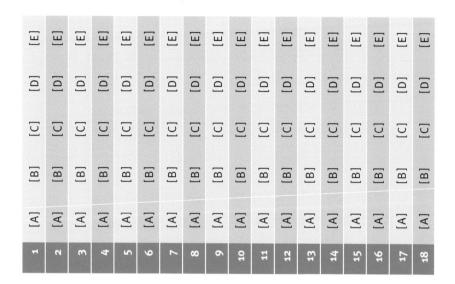

MCQs

Complete by fully filling in with pencil the lozenge corresponding to the correct answer – **True** or **False**. **T** = True and **F** = False.

	A	B	C	D	E
1	T F	T F	T F	T F	T F
2	T F	T F	T F	T F	T F
3	T F	T F	T F	T F	T F
4	T F	T F	T F	T F	T F
5	T F	T F	T F	T F	T F
6	T F	T F	T F	T F	T F
7	T F	T F	T F	T F	T F
8	T F	T F	T F	T F	T F
9	T F	T F	T F	T F	T F
10	T F	T F	T F	T F	T F
11	T F	T F	T F	T F	T F
12	T F	T F	T F	T F	T F
13	T F	T F	T F	T F	T F
14	T F	T F	T F	T F	T F
15	T F	T F	T F	T F	T F
16	T F	T F	T F	T F	T F
17	T F	T F	T F	T F	T F
18	T F	T F	T F	T F	T F
19	T F	T F	T F	T F	T F

20	[T] [F]	[T] [F]	[T] [F]	[T] [F]	[T] [F]
21	[T] [F]	[T] [F]	[T] [F]	[T] [F]	[T] [F]
22	[T] [F]	[T] [F]	[T] [F]	[T] [F]	[T] [F]
23	[T] [F]	[T] [F]	[T] [F]	[T] [F]	[T] [F]
24	[T] [F]	[T] [F]	[T] [F]	[T] [F]	[T] [F]
25	[T] [F]	[T] [F]	[T] [F]	[T] [F]	[T] [F]
26	[T] [F]	[T] [F]	[T] [F]	[T] [F]	[T] [F]
27	[T] [F]	[T] [F]	[T] [F]	[T] [F]	[T] [F]
28	[T] [F]	[T] [F]	[T] [F]	[T] [F]	[T] [F]
29	[T] [F]	[T] [F]	[T] [F]	[T] [F]	[T] [F]
30	[T] [F]	[T] [F]	[T] [F]	[T] [F]	[T] [F]
31	[T] [F]	[T] [F]	[T] [F]	[T] [F]	[T] [F]
32	[T] [F]	[T] [F]	[T] [F]	[T] [F]	[T] [F]
33	[T] [F]	[T] [F]	[T] [F]	[T] [F]	[T] [F]
34	[T] [F]	[T] [F]	[T] [F]	[T] [F]	[T] [F]
35	[T] [F]	[T] [F]	[T] [F]	[T] [F]	[T] [F]
36	[T] [F]	[T] [F]	[T] [F]	[T] [F]	[T] [F]
37	[T] [F]	[T] [F]	[T] [F]	[T] [F]	[T] [F]
38	[T] [F]	[T] [F]	[T] [F]	[T] [F]	[T] [F]
39	[T] [F]	[T] [F]	[T] [F]	[T] [F]	[T] [F]
40	[T] [F]	[T] [F]	[T] [F]	[T] [F]	[T] [F]

Index